Welcome to the Emerg

The first few months come with the biggest hurdles as there is so much to learn and experience. You will be learning how to care for and stabilize critical patients, to remain composed during emergencies and will develop "tough skin." With patience and tact, you'll become more confident and be better prepared to handle whatever comes your way.

Initially, you will work very closely with your preceptor while you learn and gain experience. Then gradually, little by little, as you building your skills, your preceptor will let you take over as they stand back and provide support when needed.

A Few Tips for Success

- **Carry a small notebook**: Take notes whenever possible and jot down questions you may have. It will serve as a reference point for you
- **Ask Every Question that comes to Mind**
- **Be Involved:** Ask your charge nurse for the critical patients. Help other nurses with critical patients. Be part of procedures.
- **Continue Learning:** Review and learn on your days off. Go over your notes. Look up any questions you may have. Ensure you understand the "why" of interventions performed.

This book came out of wanting to help new ER Nurses master the essentials of Emergency Nursing prior to going out on their own. You will truly never know everything, but if you have the basics down, you will be able to efficiently and safely care for your patients. I hope we are able to get you closer to being the best ER nurse you can be.

Target Audience

This book is for you if:

- You feel anxious when receiving a new patient
- You struggle to remember which questions to ask during assessments
- You can't figure out why certain tests or treatments were ordered by providers
- You sometimes go blank on key treatments and interventions
- You feel like you haven't mastered the basics of Emergency Nursing

While there are countless other books on emergency nursing that are very detailed and full of great information, this book focuses on helping you grasp the key foundational concepts. We cover key topics such as the ABC's and initial assessment, secondary assessment, questions to ask based on symptoms, understanding the workups, focused assessments and common emergency conditions seen in the Emergency Department.

Disclaimer

The field of medicine and emergency nursing is constantly evolving, with new research regularly updating common practices. While I strive for accuracy, the information provided in this book is based on my personal experiences and interpretations, not backed by formal research. This content reflects my perspective on various situations and is not an official source or substitute for medical advice.

This book is not intended to replace formal training or the hands-on experience you'll gain through clinical practice. Always refer to your nursing board, your organization's policies and procedures, and the guidance of your preceptors and educators. Additionally, this information is not a substitute for advice or care from your primary healthcare provider and is intended for entertainment purposes only.

I have shared my experiences to avoid plagiarism. However, if you believe I have unintentionally infringed on any material, please reach out so we can address it appropriately—whether that means giving credit or removing the content.

Table of Contents

Contents

Purpose of Emergency Department and Role of the ER Nurse

The main purpose of the Emergency Department is to identify, prioritize and treat life threatening conditions. Based on a patients symptoms and presentation, providers (Doctors, physician assistants, nurse practitioners) will form a list of the possible causes, known as the "differential diagnosis." This list will guide the workup and treatment.

Nurses are commonly the first to come in contact with patients when they arrive to the ER. As a result, nurses perform triage where they assign an acuity level to patients. This acuity level often dictates how fast patients get seen by a provider, making it essential for an emergency nurse to have great assessment skills in order to quickly detect potential life threatening conditions.

In addition to triage, based on what the provider orders, nurses obtain laboratory studies, place intravenous catheters, transport patients to radiology/imaging, administer medications, perform interventions, closely monitor and advocate for patients, think critically and efficiently and promptly communicate with the providers as needed. We even serve as the last final check to ensure ordered interventions are appropriate for our patients, keeping their best interests in mind.

Patient Arrival: Initial Impression & ABC's

First and foremost, you will be proactive, not reactive. Your rooms will have all the necessary equipment and supplies needed for an emergency. These include:

- Bag Valve Masks (adult and pediatric)
- Suction and Oxygen Equipment
- Supplies needed to connect the patient onto the monitor

When your patient arrives:
- Obtain an initial impression
- Focus on the ABC's (Airway, Breathing, Circulation)
- Get your patient on the monitor
- Gather pertinent history
- Prepare to place an IV if needed.

Initial Impression

The initial impression, or visual assessment, involves quickly scanning the patient to gather easy to see visual information about their overall condition. Essentially, at a glance, you are trying to see **how sick a patient looks**.

- **General Mentation (Neuro)**
  - Are they awake and alert?
  - Somnolent, drowsy or easily falling asleep?
- **Circulation and Perfusion**
  - Skin color? Cool clammy skin? Diaphoretic and pale? Mottled?
  - Peripheral Edema?
- **Breathing**
  - Visible respiratory distress? Rapid breathing?
  - Use of accessory muscles? Audible wheezing or stridor?
- **Discomfort and Pain**
  - Grimacing or Guarding a specific area?

The initial impression is useful because at a glance, it allows you to determine if a patient "looks" sick and if so, they can be prioritized.

Airway Breathing Circulation

A common misconception is that the ABC's are performed one at a time. While the ABCs are approached systematically, many things happen simultaneously. For example, while connecting to the cardiac monitor, you can ask questions regarding their visit. If they are speaking and breathing without issues, you note their 'Airway' and 'Breathing' are intact. If you are having airway or breathing issues, you won't be speaking in nice calm sentences. On the other hand, when a patient is in respiratory distress, you will place them on oxygen, on the cardiac monitor and place an IV, while the provider is moving down the ABC's. Everyone is working as a team to help stabilize the patient.

The ABCs systematic method guides healthcare providers including nurses in quickly identifying and treating conditions that compromise oxygenation, ventilation, and perfusion.

1) **Airway: Assessment and Interventions**
   a) Assessment: Evaluate for Airway Obstruction
      i) If speaking, the airway is open.
      ii) Swelling/Edema, Strider, Gurgling sounds or Hoarseness of the voice
      iii) Secretions, Vomitus or Foreign Body
   b) Interventions
      i) Position Maneuvers
         (1) Head Tilt Chin Lift
         (2) If concern for cervical/spinal trauma, Perform Jaw Thrust
      ii) Airway Adjuncts
         (1) Oropharyngeal Airway
            (a) Only if no gag reflex present in comatose patient
         (2) Nasopharyngeal Airway
            (a) Only when there is no facial trauma
         (3) Suction
         (4) Oxygen Administration
            (a) Non Rebreather Reservoir Mask (NRB)
            (b) Bag Valve Mask (BVM)
         (5) Endotracheal Intubation
         (6) Cricothyroidotomy

2) **Breathing Assessment and Interventions**

a) Assessment
   i) Observe Rate, Depth and Use of Accessory Muscles
   ii) Lung Sounds and Symmetry of Chest Rise
   iii) Spo2
b) Interventions
   i) Oxygen
     (1) NRB
     (2) BVM
       (a) Ventilating the patient (providing breaths-observe for chest rise) if no spontaneous or ineffective breaths are present
   ii) High Flow, Noninvasive Ventilation (Bipap/Cpap)
   iii) Needle Decompression and Chest Tubes
   iv) Intubation

3) **Circulation**
a) Assessment for adequate perfusion
   i) Capillary Refill, Pulses, Heart Rate, Skin Color, Blood Pressure, Mentation, ECG
   ii) Locate Sites of Bleeding
b) Interventions
   i) Fluid Administration, Blood Products, Vasopressors, Medications to help with oncotic pressure such as Albumin
   ii) Tourniquet, Vessel Ligation
   iii) CPR and ACLS Algorithms

4) **Disability**
a) Assessment
   i) Level of Consciousness, Orientation Status, GCS
   ii) Pupils and Glucose
   iii) Motor and Sensory Function
b) Interventions
   i) Radiology to Pinpoint areas of damage
   ii) Glucose Administration
   iii) Intubation for airway protection r/t decreased mentation

Protect the C-Spine when performing airway maneuvers.

Secondary Assessment

The secondary assessment is a comprehensive evaluation conducted after the initial stabilization in order to identify injuries or issues that may have been missed. It focuses on obtaining a detailed medical history, performing a head-to-toe physical examination, obtaining diagnostic studies and laboratory tests.

1) **Gathering Medical History**
   a) Helps gain an insight into the patient's overall health and can help identify causes of the patient's current condition
   b) **SAMPLE Mnemonic**
      i) S: **Signs and Symptoms**
         (1) Chief complaint and presenting symptoms. Obtain information about the onset, duration, location, severity, and associated factors of their symptoms.
      ii) A: **Allergies**
         (1) Inquire about any known allergies, including medications, food, environmental, or other allergens. Document the type of reaction.
      iii) M: **Medication Use**
         (1) Ask the patient about their current medications, including prescription, over-the-counter, and herbal supplements. Document the name, dosage, frequency. Ask about compliance and any recent changes to their medications.
      iv) P: **Past Medical History**
         (1) Diagnosed Conditions
         (2) Surgeries
         (3) Drug/Alcohol/Smoking
         (4) Recent Hospitalizations
         (5) Pertinent Family History
      v) L: **Last Oral Intake or Last Meal**
         (1) Determine the patient's last oral intake of food, fluids, or medications. Document the time and type of intake, especially if the patient may require sedation, anesthesia, or surgical procedures.
      vi) **Events**
         (1) Ask about the events leading up to their current condition. Gather information about any trauma,

environmental exposures, activities, or lifestyle factors that may be relevant to their condition.

2) **Repeat Set of Vital Signs**
   a) Repeating vital signs allows nurses to monitor the patient's response to interventions and assess for any changes in their condition. Vital signs provide valuable insights into the patient's physiological status, helping nurses identify signs of improvement, deterioration, or instability.
   b) Heart Rate, Blood Pressure, Respiratory Rate, Spo2, Temperature and Pain
      i) **Heart Rate**: High or Low can cause a patient to become unstable
         (1) Tachycardia: Can be a sign of pain, fever, shock, or cardiac issues.
         (2) Bradycardia: May indicate issues such as cardiac conduction issues, hypothermia and medication side effects. Any heart rate <40 should be taken seriously despite a "stable blood pressure."
      ii) **Blood Pressure:** High or Low can lead to perfusion issues and organ damage
         (1) Hypertension: Can indicate underlying cardiovascular disease, renal dysfunction, stress and poor compliance with medications.
         (2) Hypotension: May signify hypovolemia and shock (different types of shock)
      iii) **Respiratory Rate**
         (1) Tachypnea: May be a sign of respiratory distress, hypoxia, pain, anxiety, or metabolic acidosis.
         (2) Bradypnea: Can indicate drug overdose, central nervous system depression, or respiratory failure.
      iv) **Spo2**
         (1) Hypoxemia: Can be due to respiratory failure, pneumonia, asthma, airway obstruction and countless respiratory issues.
      v) **Temperature**
         (1) Hyperthermia: May indicate infection, inflammation, or heat-related illness

(2) Hypothermia: Can result from exposure to cold environments, shock, or other issues.

3) **Head to Toe Examination**
   a) A more thorough examination is necessary to ensure nothing is missed. Ensure to turn the patient and assess everything. Go through each body system: Neuro, Cardiac, Resp, GI and so forth.
   b) We will go more in depth on assessments and how to perform in the later chapters.

4) **Diagnostic Studies and Laboratory Tests**
   a) Can help identify underlying medical conditions or injuries that may not be immediately apparent during the initial assessment.
   b) Can confirm or rule out suspected diagnoses
      i) For example, imaging studies such as X-rays can help confirm ortho issues like fractures and dislocations, while CTs can help confirm internal issues like gallstones and pulmonary embolisms. Laboratory tests can confirm infectious diseases, metabolic imbalances, or organ dysfunction. We will review labs in a later chapter.
   c) Can help gauge disease severity: how sick are they
      i) For example, a high lactate is known to a be sign of poor tissue perfusion and poor outcomes if no interventions are performed while an ABG can help assess the severity of respiratory conditions by looking at the PaO2 and PaCo2.

5) **Recognition of Abnormal Findings and Prompt Communication**
   a) As the primary nurse, one of your roles is to keep track of assessment findings and results, and promptly communicating/relaying when there is an abnormal finding.
   b) For example, if on the repeat set of vitals after the initial stabilization you start noticing a trend of the BP going lower and lower, or the heart rate going higher and higher, or if the potassium level is 6.8 or even the patient's mentation changing.
      i) You will need to continuously be on the lookout for abnormal findings and promptly communicate. Of course, perform a good assessment so that when you speak to your provider you are able to paint the whole picture of the situation and provide a good SBAR

Triage

Triage is a process where patients are categorized based on the potential or severity of their condition. Categories typically range from "immediate" or "resuscitation" for patients requiring immediate life-saving interventions, to "non-urgent" for those with minor complaints or stable conditions that can safely wait for evaluation and treatment. It boils down to, **does this patient need immediate interventions or can they wait?**

Factors that are assessed include:

1) **Chief Complaint with Signs and Symptoms**
   a) Chest Pain
      i) Can be a symptom of various serious conditions like myocardial infarction and pulmonary embolisms (Countless other reasons)
   b) Shortness of Breath
      i) Can indicate respiratory distress or compromise due to conditions such as pneumonia, asthma or COPD exacerbation, pulmonary edema, or pneumothorax. (Countless other reasons)
   c) Altered Mental Status
      i) Can be a sign of neurological dysfunction or systemic illness, including hypoglycemia, stroke or sepsis. (Countless other reasons)
   d) Trauma
      i) Patients with severe trauma, such as motor vehicle accidents, falls from high heights, stab wounds, gun shot wounds, require immediate attention to manage life-threatening injuries.
   e) Stroke Symptoms
      i) Patients with sudden-onset focal neurological deficits, such as facial droop, arm weakness, slurred speech, unilateral numbness.
   f) Fever in Pediatric Patients
      i) Can be a sign of a serious underlying infection so make them a priority as pediatric patients may have limited or underdeveloped immune systems

2) **Vital Signs**
   a) Vital signs help assess a patients overall status. Abnormal vital signs, such as tachycardia, hypotension, tachypnea, or hypoxemia, indicate a serious issue that needs to be addressed. This further validates a need to place a patient as a higher priority to receive attention and interventions.
   b) For example, if a patient presents with shortness of breath with a respiratory rate of 34 and an SPO2 of 85%, it warrants the triage nurse to place the patient as a higher priority, immediately notifying the charge nurse of the need for this patient to be placed in a room for immediate stabilization interventions. Another example would be if a family member brings a patient for Altered Mental Status and decreased PO intake with a heart rate of 150's and bp of 84/55. This would require the patient to receive immediate attention.

3) **Potential for Deterioration and Time Sensitive Conditions**
   a) Stroke Symptoms
   b) Anaphylaxis and Allergic Reactions
   c) Suicidal and Homocidal Ideation
   d) ACS (Stemi, Nstemi, Unstable Angina)
   e) Conditions that are time sensitive such as these should be assigned with a triage level that places them at a higher priority.

4) **Risk Factors**
   a) Age
      i) Neonates, children and the elderly should be placed as a priority due to the potential for serious injury.
   b) Medical History
      i) Diabetes, hypertension, known heart disease, increased cholesterol, smoker, or immunosuppression, place the patient at an increased risk for complications.
   c) Medications
      i) Patients presenting with issues of high risk medications like blood thinners, insulins, opioids, immunosuppressants and pediatric medications should be assessed more rapidly to ascertain the risk for serious injury.
   d) Recent procedures and surgeries
      i) Recent surgeries or invasive procedures may be at increased risk for complications such as infection and bleeding.

e) Social Risk Factors
   i) Alcohol Use
   ii) Smoking History
   iii) Drug Use

Putting all the details and information together is the key. For example, an elderly patient with chest pain and stable vitals will be assigned a higher priority than a patient in their 20's with the same chief complaint and vital signs. **To simplify it, again, can this patient wait to be seen?** should they wait to be seen? Should they skip the line? **Should they receive immediate care?** Should they be seen first in the fast track area by a provider? Or **should they be placed in a resuscitation room** for immediate critical care and life saving interventions?

Emergency Severity Index

There are many triaging algorithms used in Emergency Departments. We will only cover the Emergency Severity Index (ESI) here. If your ER uses a different system, please become familiar with it. Although, many principles are interchangeable. The Emergency Severity Index (ESI) is a five-level triage algorithm used to prioritize patients in the emergency department (ED) based on the acuity of their condition and the anticipated resource needs.

1) **Level 1 – Immediate**
   a) Patients with life-threatening conditions requiring immediate interventions. These patients should be seen immediately.
   b) Examples: Cardiac and respiratory arrest, severe trauma, active hemorrhage, acute myocardial infarction, stroke with neurological deficits, severe respiratory distress.

2) **Level 2 – Emergent**
   a) Patients with potentially life-threatening conditions.These patients are unstable and may deteriorate without prompt medical attention. These patients should be seen by a provider within 10 minutes.
   b) Examples: Chest pain with suspected ACS, asthma exacerbation, moderate trauma and so forth. These patients will have unstable vital signs.

3) **Level 3 – Urgent**

a) Patients with stable vital signs, do require prompt assessment and intervention, however, the condition is not life threatening at that moment in time. These patients should be seen within 30 minutes.
b) Examples: Abdominal pain, asthma or copd without change in vital signs, possible fractures, skin infections like cellulitis.

4) Level - Less Urgent
a) Stable patients, can wait for up to 1 hour. No life threatening conditions.
b) Examples: Lacerations requiring sutures, sprain or strain, minor burns, or mild pain.

5) Level 5 - Non Urgent
a) Do not require immediate attention, no life threatening condition, may wait for an extended period of time.
b) Examples: Cold symptoms, medication refills, suture removal.

The ESI algothrym is designed to efficiently categorize patients according to their level of urgency, ensuring that those with the most critical conditions receive timely care.

Guide to Questioning

It is very difficult in the beginning of your ER career to know what questions to ask when assessing as the questions change by chief complaint and patient. Below is a mini guide as to what questions you should be asking. With time, these will be second nature, and you may develop a better flow or list of more concise questions to ask.

There are questions that you will ask every patient and to make it easy to remember, it is the SAMPLE mnemonic we discussed earlier. We will also ask the PQRST questions.

SAMPLE (Symptoms, Allergies, Medications, Past Medical History, Last Intake, Events)

1) **Allergies**
    a)   "Do you have any allergies to medications or foods?"

2) **Medications**
    a)   "What medications are you currently taking?"

3) **Past Medical History**
    a)   "Have you been diagnosed with any medical conditions in the past such as high blood pressure, diabetes, high cholesterol?"
    b)   "Have you had any recent surgeries or hospitalizations?"
    c)   "Do you smoke? Drink alcohol regularly? Or do any illicit drugs?"
        i)   When asking about illicit drug use, I find it helpful to say "We are asking to be better able to care for you, we are not the cops, we are not going to report you. Again, it is so we can have a clear picture of everything and be better able to help you."

4) **Last Intake**
    a)   When was the last time you ate or drank anything? What was it?"
        i)   I'm only asking this question when I anticipate a patient requiring sedation whether for a bedside procedure or surgery. In the ER, I will ask for patients who have fractures as they may

undergo a conscious sedation to get the bone back in
alignment. (Remind them not to eat or drink anything?

5) Events
   a) "Can you tell me what happened?"

<u>PQRST</u> (*P*rovocation/*P*alliative, *Q*uality, *R*egion/*R*adiation,
*S*everity, *T*iming)

1) Provocation / Palliative
   a) "What makes your pain worse?"
   b) "What makes it better?"

2) Quality
   a) "How does your pain feel?" "Can you describe your pain?"
      i) Is it sharp, dull, aching, burning or throbbing?

3) Region / Radiation
   a) "Where is your pain?"
   b) "Does your pain radiate anywhere?"

4) Severity
   a) "On a scale of 0 to 10, with 0 being no pain and 10 being the worst
       pain imaginable, how would you rate your pain?"

5) Timing
   a) "When did the pain start? Is it constant or does it come and go?"

***<u>*You need to ask the SAMPLE questions to every patient. The PQRST
to every patient with pain.</u>***

Complaint Based Questions

1) Chest Pain
   a) Where is the pain located? Can you point to it?
   b) Can you describe the pain?
   c) How long have you had this pain?
   d) Did anything trigger this pain? What were you doing when it started?
   e) Does the pain radiate anywhere?
   f) How bad is the pain on a scale from 0 to 10?
   g) Have you had pain like this before? What was done?
   h) Are you having any other symptoms like dizziness, shortness of breath or nausea? Other symptoms you can ask about include weakness, cough, swelling in the legs, distended abdomen.
   i) Then of course, as the SAMPLE questions.

2) Shortness of Breath
   a) How long have you had shortness of breath?
   b) Is the SOB constant or does it come and go? What makes it better? What makes it worse?
   c) What were you doing when the SOB started?
   d) Are you having any other symptoms?
   e) Have you had any recent surgeries or been immobile for a long time such as a long car ride or flight?
   f) Has this happened before? Do you have a history of heart or lung issues? Do you smoke?
   g) Then of course, as the SAMPLE questions.
      i) Do note, that for your respiratory patients who are in active distress, you will be performing interventions first then once they are stabilized will be asking the questions. Like asthma exacerbation patients will most likely not be able to speak to you from how short of breath they are.

3) Abdominal Pain
   a) Where is your pain? Can you point to your pain?
   b) How long have you had the pain? Was it sudden or gradual?
   c) Did you eat anything that could have caused this pain?
   d) How would you describe the pain?
   e) Does the pain radiate anywhere?

f) What makes the pain better? What makes the pain worse?
g) Any changes in bowel habits or urination? Does it hurt to pee?
h) Are you having any other symptoms?
   i) Like fevers, nausea, vomiting, diarrhea, constipation, bleeding from the rectum or when vomiting?
i) Has this happened before? What was done? Prior GI issues, diagnoses or surgeries?
j) For women of child bearing age: Any chance of pregnancy? When was your last menstrual cycle? Any vaginal bleeding or spotting?
k) Then of course, as the SAMPLE questions.

4) **Motor Vehicle Accident**
   a) How fast were you going?
   b) Were you wearing a seatbelt? Separation from vehicle?
   c) Did the airbags go off?
   d) Did you lose consciousness?
   e) Mechanism
      i) Direction of Impact: Struck head on, rear ended, struck on drivers side of passenger side
      ii) Position in vehicle: Driver, passenger, back seat etc
      iii) Vehicle damage: Roll over, Extensive damage, minor accident, vehicle intrusion, dash damage etc
   f) Where is your pain?
   g) These patients require a thorough initial stabilization and secondary assessment to ensure nothing is missed. Looking at the head, neck, back, chest, abdo, pelvis, long bones, deformities and so forth. Ensuring no injury is missed. Checking for internal injuries and bleeding, checking for sensation and strength. Vital signs. And constant monitoring and reevaluation.
   h) Then of course, as the SAMPLE questions.

5) **Syncope and Loss of Consciousness**
   a) What happened before it? Any Chest pain, dizziness, sob or headache prior to event?
   b) What were you doing when it happened?
   c) Did anyone witness it? What did they notice? How long were you unconscious?
   d) Did you hit your head? Any head neck or back pain? Loss of sensation or strength?

e) Has it happened before? What was done, what were you told?
f) Are you having any symptoms right now? Cp, sob, dizziness, palpitations, headache etc
g) After you regained consciousness, did you feel confused or were you back to normal mentally?
h) Have you been eating and drinking water?
i) Then of course, as the SAMPLE questions.

6) **Back Pain**
   a) Where is your back pain?
   b) When did it start?
   c) Does it radiate anywhere? Down just one leg?
      i) Any numbness, tingling, or weakness in the legs?
   d) Can you describe the pain?
   e) Out of 10, how bad is it?
   f) Any issues urinating or with your bowels?
   g) Does anything make it worse or better?
      i) Did you take any over the counter meds, have you rested, have they helped?
   h) Has this happened before and what were you told?
   i) Any trauma?
   j) What were you doing prior to it starting, did you lift anything heavy or bend wrong?
   k) Then of course, as the SAMPLE questions.

7) **Seizures**
   a) Was it witness? If so, what did they noticed?
   b) Did you have an auro prior to?
   c) Do you have a history of seizures? Have they happened before? When was the last one?
   d) Do you take medications for it? Which one? Dose?
   e) Have you been taking your meds? Has there been a change in your meds?
   f) Did you urinate on yourself or bite your tongue during?
   g) Are you feeling confused? (Ask the orientation questions)
   h) Ask trauma questions if they fell down (Head neck or back pain? Sensation? Strength? Etc)
   i) Any recent sickness or head trauma?
   j) Then of course, as the SAMPLE questions.

8) Suicidal Ideation
   a) Are you feeling like hurting yourself right now?
   b) Is there anything making you feel this way? Any stressful events happening?
   c) Do you feel like hurting others?
   d) Are you having any hallucinations? Are you seeing or hearing any strange voices or figures?
   e) Do you have a plan in place?
   f) Has this ever happened to you before? Have you ever tried to hurt yourself in the past?
   g) Have you been drinking or using drugs today?
   h) Then of course, as the SAMPLE questions.

9) Asthma Exacerbation
   a) How long have you been short of breath?
   b) Did anything trigger it?
   c) Have you been using your inhaler? How often per day?
      i) Any recent changes in your asthma meds?
   d) How often do you have to come to the ER?
   e) Have you ever been intubated or had to go to the ICU for your asthma?
   f) Then of course, as the SAMPLE questions.

10) GI Bleed
   a) How long have you been bleeding for?
   b) Rectal bleeding or with vomiting?
   c) What color is it? Bright red or black?
   d) For rectal bleeding, is the whole toilet bowl red, streaks or only red on the toilet paper when you wipe?
   e) For vomiting blood, how often? How much? (You can ask, How many cups?)
   f) Do you take blood thinners?
   g) Has this happened before and what was done? What were you told?
   h) History of esophageal varices?
   i) Then of course, as the SAMPLE questions.

i) Associated symptoms, abdominal surgeries, meds like blood thinners, diagnosed GI issues, alcohol and liver issues and so forth.

11) Congestive Heart Failure Exacerbation
a) Do you take diuretics? (Do you take water pills?)
   i) Did you notice that you gained weight?
b) Have you been taking your medications?
c) How long have you been short of breath for? How long for fatigue, leg swelling, feeling like drowning while laying flat?
d) What is your ejection fraction? (Do you know the percentage of how good your heart is working?)
e) Then of course, as the SAMPLE questions.

12) Hyperglycemia and DKA
a) What medications do you take? Have you been taking them?
b) What is your sugar typically at home?
c) Did you recently binge drink?
d) Any recent infections or illnesses?
e) Increase in thirst? Urination? Nausea? Abdominal Pain?
f) Then of course, as the SAMPLE questions.

13) Allergic Reaction
a) Has this happened before and what was done?
b) Do you know what could have triggered it? Any new lotions, shampoos, soap, detergents?
   i) What were you doing or where were you when it started?
c) Have you ever developed breathing issues? Have you ever had swelling of your tongue or throat?
d) Are you feeling sob or like your throat is closing?
e) How long have you had these symptoms? (Rash hives etc)
f) What are your known allergies?
g) Then of course, as the SAMPLE questions.

14) Stroke Symptoms
a) How long have you had these symptoms? When were you last normal? What time did these symptoms start?
b) What specific symptoms are you having?

      i)   Facial droop, slurring, numbness, tingling, weakness, coordination issues?
- c) Check blood sugar to rule out hypoglycemia.
- d) Has this happened before? Did it go away by itself? What was done?
- e) If within window for thrombolytics, ensure no contraindications such as recent head trauma, blood thinner use, recent surgeries, recent stroke, brain lesions, active bleeding etc
- f) Then of course, as the SAMPLE questions.

15) Pediatric Fever
- a) How long have they had the fever?
- b) Did you give any medications today? Which ones? How much and how long ago?
- c) Any sick siblings or other family members?
- d) How are they acting?
- e) Are they eating and drinking? How many bowel movements and urinations per day?
- f) Do they have all of their vaccinations? Any recent vaccinations?
- g) Ask about whether the patient has had a cough, runny nose, pulling at their ear, pain with urination, or pain in their abdomen. Any wounds?
- h) How high has the fever been at home?
- i) Then of course, as the SAMPLE questions.

Vasopressors

Vasopressors, also commonly known as pressors, are potent medications that **constrict blood vessels**, ultimately, increasing blood pressure with the goal of restoring tissue perfusion in very hypotensive patients. Besides vasoconstriction, they can also affect **heart contractility**, and **heart rate**. Epinephrine also affects the lungs.

1) Alpha Receptors (Found in blood vessels- vascular smooth muscle cells)
   a) Cause Vasoconstriction when stimulated, with an ultimate increase in blood pressure.
2) Beta 1 Receptors (Found in the heart)
   a) Cause an increase in the strength of contraction of the heart (positive inotropic effect) and an increase in heart heart rate when stimulated (positive chronotropic effect).
3) Beta 2 Receptors (Found in bronchial smooth muscle of the lungs)
   a) Cause bronchodilation when stimulated
   b) It can also cause vasodilation
4) V1 Receptors (Found in smooth muscle cells of blood vessels)
   a) Cause vasoconstriction when stimulated

Caution with Vasopressors
Although vasopressors can save a patient's life, they come with many possible and deadly complications.
   1. *Never Bolus vasopressors*

Complications
   • Increase Risk for Arrhythmias
   • Cardiac, Organ and Periphery Ischemia
   • Tissue Necrosis from Extravasation
   • Rapid Increase in Bp

Now lets talk about specific vasopressors and why they are used in shock (to help increase the bp and ultimately help increase the perfusion to organs).

Norepinephrine (Levophed)

- Potent Alpha Agonist with *Slight* Beta 1
  - Increase blood pressure through vasoconstriction
  - Help the heart squeeze/contract a little better and faster
- **Can be started peripherally in emergencies** (Peripheral infusion should be no more than 1-2 hours. Advocate for a central line).
- Known as the "**workhorse**" vasopressor because it is often the first line vasopressor used for many issues.
  - Pressor of choice for septic shock. It can also be used as the first line agent for neurogenic, cardiogenic and obstructive shock when needed.
    - Also used in hypovolemic shock, however, *only when the patient has been appropriately volume resuscitated (fluids, blood products).*
- Onset: within 1-2 minutes
- Concentration: 4mg in 250ml of NS (it can also be 8mg in 250, or up to 16mg in 250)
- Range and Titration Range from facility to facility (Fill out with your own facilities protocol)
  - Start Dose:
  - Titrate By:
  - Range/Max:

Vasopressin

- Potent V1 Agonist
  - Increases BP
- Second Line Agent in Septic Shock, added on after Norepinephrine(Levophed)
  - After constantly titrating Levophed up and are near the max dose, notify the provider and suggest vasopressin be added. You'll notice a big difference in the bp and in perfusion.
- Onset: Up to 15 minutes
- *Do not Titrate*
  - Start it and leave it alone
  - Rate: 0.04U/min
- Concentration
  - 20 Units in 100ml of NS (or 50 Units in 250Ml of NS)

Epinephrine

- Alpha, Beta 1, Beta 2
  - Vasoconstriction, Increases HR and contraction, Bronchodilation
- Vasopressor of choice with anaphylactic shock and in shock states where the heart rate is low (bradycardia patients) as it will help bring the heart rate and bp up together
  - Added on after Levophed and vasopressin in septic patients
- Onset: within 1 minute
- Concentration: 1mg in 250 ml or 4mg in 250 ml
- Range and Titration Range from facility to facility (Fill out with your own facilities protocol)
  - Start Dose:
  - Titrate By:
  - Range/Max:
- Dirty Epinephrine Drip
  - In Emergencies when the patient is about to code, I've had providers order a "Dirty Epi Drip." Essentially you get 1mg of epi(an amp from the crash cart), and you inject it into a 1L NS bag(label it of course). This 1L of NS with 1mg of Epi is then administered "wide open" to the patient.
    - The point of this is to give you enough time to stabilize the patient and then place them on an actual drip.
    - You should not be doing this unless your provider explicitly states they want this and your preceptor is with you.
- Push Dose Epi
  - You should also be aware that your provider may admin a push dose of Epinephrine to your patient in an emergengy to bring their bp up so they dont code.. It will be approximately **10 mcg.** It is not in our scope to administer this but it is nice to know about it.
- Epinephrine is used in a variety of ways including during Cardiopulmonary Arrest, as a Push Dose Pressor, as a Vasopressor and even in laceration repairs.

Phenylephrine (Neosynephrine)

- Pure Alpha
  - Only vasoconstriction

- o Be mindful that if you only increase the BP, if too high, the body may try to bring the BP down by decreasing the heart rate. (Can cause bradycardia so be careful with bradycardic patients)
- Typically an add on vasopressor when the others have not worked. It is also used with anaphylaxis to help vasoconstrict and bring the BP back up.
- Onset: within 1 minute
- Concentration: 20mg in 250ml or 50mg in 250 ml of NS
- Can also be used as a push dose vasopressor just like Epinephrine
  - o Its typical dose for adults will be 100-200 mcg. Just like with Epi, it is not in our scope to push this, it must be the provider.
- Range and Titration Range from facility to facility (Fill out with your own facilities protocol)
  - o Start Dose:
  - o Titrate By:
  - o Range/Max:

- ***Dopamine***
  - o Alpha, B1, and Effects on the Kidneys
    - ▪ Dose dependent. It can be difficult to know what it effects it will have
      - For this reason, at least in the ER, it's not really used, since we can use levophed and epinephrine, and we know what we are getting with those two.
    - ▪ Typically on lower doses it increases blood flow to the kidneys and on higher doses it causes vasoconstriction and an increase in heart/contraction
  - o Onset: within 5 minutes
  - o Concentration: 400mg in 250ml of NS
  - o Range and Titration Range from facility to facility (Fill out with your own facilities protocol)
    - ▪ Start Dose:
    - ▪ Titrate By:
    - ▪ Range/Max:

Dobutamine

- Beta 1, Beta 2 and Alpha Agonist
  - Primary effect is on Beta 1, especially on **helping the heart contract** better
  - Since beta 2 can also cause vasodilation, it often counteracts the effects of Alpha. It can, at times, cause more vasodilation and lead to hypotension after starting the infusion.
- It's main use will be in Cardiogenic Shock from heart failure
- Onset: Up to 10 minutes
- Concentration: 500mg in 250ml of NS
- Range and Titration Range from facility to facility (Fill out with your own facilities protocol)
  - Start Dose:
  - Titrate By:
  - Range/Max:

General Vasopressor Tips

- Start norepinephrine peripherally in emergency situations!
- Pressors are typically compatible with each other.
- Always have your next bag ready to go! Never let the bag run dry.
- You must learn how to make a Levophed, an Epi and a vasopressin drip for emergency situations or when pharmacy is not available.
- You do not titrate vasopressin.
- They all suck in severe acidosis, except vasopressin.
- Tidy Up! Label all your lines at the patient and by the pump!
- Do not bolus! Ever. (After titrating, give them time to work)
- Set your BP's to take Q5Minutes, or quicker! So you can keep an eye on how the patient is responding.
- If you are starting a second pressor, you better be asking for an Arterial Line to closely monitor the BP.
- Ask for a central line.
- Keep an eye on mcg/min vs mcg/kg/min.

ACLS Medications

- **Cardiac Arrest**
  - *Epinephrine*
    - Cardiac Arrest (Asystole, PEA, Vfib, Vtach without a pulse)
      - Given during cardiac arrest to improve coronary and cerebral perfusion. As a vasoconstrictor and inotropic agent, it helps improve the chances of obtain ROSC (Return of Spontaneous Circulation)
      - Dose: 1 mg every 3-5 minutes IV/IO

  - *Calcium Chloride*
    - Calcium plays an important role in myocardial cell membrane stability and contractility.
    - It is given during cardiac arrest when certain issues are suspected such as Hyperkalemia, Hypocalcemia, and calcium channel blocker overdose.
      - Hyperkalemia: High levels of potassium irritate the heart which can lead to deadly arrhythmias. Calcium stabilizes cardiac cell membranes.
      - Hypocalcemia: Given to replace the needed calcium.
      - Calcium Channel Blocker OD: Calcium chloride helps counteract the effects on cardiac and smooth muscle cells by helping restore cardiac conduction, cardiac contractility, and prevent the vasodilation effects.
    - Adult Dose: 1g IV/IO (10ml of a 10% calcium chloride solution)

  - *Sodium Bicarbonate*
    - During cardiac arrest it is given to help treat the severe metabolic acidosis since acidosis impairs

cardiac function and cellular metabolism. By counteracting the acidosis, we are helping improve the chances of obtaining ROSC (Return of Spontaneous Circulation)
- Adult Dose: 50mEq (50 ml of an 8.4% Sodium Bicarb)

- ### *Amiodarone*
  - An antiarrhythmic used during cardiac arrest for ventricular fibrillation and ventricular tachycardia without a pulse.
  - Prolongs the action potential and refractory period of cardiac cells. Vfib and Vtach without a pulse are essentially rhythms where the ventricles are very excitable and irritable, by prolonging the action potential and the refractory period, it helps calm down cardiac cells (less irritable and less excitable).
  - Adult Dose: 300mg IV, then if needed, a repeat 150mg.
    - Note that if ROSC is obtain, an infusion of amiodarone should be initiated.

- ### *Lidocaine*
  - An antiarrhythmic used during cardiac arrest for ventricular fibrillation and ventricular tachycardia without a pulse.
  - It blocks sodium channels in cardiac cells which help slow down conduction and ultimately stabilize cardiac cell membranes as a result.
    - Remember that during the action potential, there is depolarization and repolarization. Depolarization is started by the influx of sodium, and the faster this occurs, the more excitable or irritable the cell can be. By slowing it down, you are essentially calming it down.
  - Adult Dose: 1 to 1.5 mg/kg IV/IO then if needed a repeat of 0.5 to 0.75 mg/kg IV/IO

- *Magnesium Sulfate*
  - Used in cardiac arrest to help treat torsades de pointes (Polymorphic ventricular tachycardia)
  - Magnesium is essential in helping cell membrane ion channels work well and when there is an imbalance, Polymorphic ventricular tachycardia results
  - Adult Dose: 2 g
    - If successful, an infusion/drip of magnesium should be started.

- *Narcan*
  - Reversal of suspected opioid overdose
    - Opioid overdose will result in respiratory depression and ultimate arrest if left untreated
  - Adult Dose: 0.4 to 2 mg IV/IO/IN/IM (If there is no pulse, you will be doing 2mg IVP)
    - If successful, an infusion/drip should be started.
  - High doses often lead to flash pulmonary edema and as a result a poor outcome.

- *Dextrose*
  - Treatment of hypoglycemia
  - Adult Dose: 25g (50 ml of a 50% dextrose solution) IV
    - If successful, continue to monitor glucose levels closely and if needed an infusion/drip should be started of D5 or D10

- *IV Fluids*
  - Normal Saline or Lactated Ringers
  - Used during cardiac arrest when needed to replenish intravascular volume. This can help improve perfusion and as a result increase the chances of obtaining ROSC.

- Other ACLS Medications
  - **Atropine**
    - Used in Symptomatic Bradycardia. It blocks parasympathetic stimulation of the heart (blocks the vagus nerve) and as a result improves conduction through the AV node.
    - Adult Dose: 1mg every 3-5 minutes, max of 3mg
    - Note that atropine may not be effective in 3rd degree AV blocks. May still be ordered to give it by the provider, however, you should be preparing more adequate treatments like Transcutaneous Pacing
  - **Adenosine**
    - Used in Supraventricular Tachycardia (SVT)
    - It has a very short half life of 10 seconds and works by blocking conduction through the AV node. This helps stop the rapid rhythm and allows the SA node to take over (as it should).
    - Given as a rapid IV push followed by a 20ml NS rapid flush to ensure it reaches the heart as again it has a very short half life of 10 seconds.
    - Adult Dose: 6mg IVP, if not successful followed by 12mg IVP. Then a third dose if needed of 12mg IVP.

H's and T's: Reversible Causes of Cardiac Arrest

The reversible causes of cardia arrest. Addressing these reversible causes improve the chances of obtaining ROSC (Return of Spontaneous Circulation)

1. **H's:**
   - **Hypovolemia**: -> Intravenous Fluids
   - **Hypoxia**: -> Oxygen via BVM or ET Tube
   - Hydrogen Ions (**Acidosis**): -> Sodium Bicarbonate
   - **Hypo-/Hyperkalemia:** -> Calcium Chloride and Sodium Bicarbonate
   - **Hypothermia:** -> Warm the patient as needed
2. **T's:**
   - **Tension Pneumothorax**: -> Needle Decompression or Chest Tube
   - **Tamponade** (Cardiac): -> Pericardiocentesis
   - **Toxins**: -> Sodium Bicarbonate, Calcium Chloride and indicated antidotes
   - **Thrombosis** (Coronary or Pulmonary): -> Thrombolytic
   - **Trauma**: -> Control bleeding, Blood Products, Surgical Interventions

Rhythms and their Treatments

The following are supposed to be quick and simple reference points for the deadly rhythms you will encounter. By no means is it comprehensive, but it should serve as a quick simple reference of key treatments.

- **CPR**: Maintains cerebral and coronary perfusion
  - If you defibrillate, immediately resume CPR for 2 minutes because even if the rhythm converted out of Ventricular Fibrillation or Pulseless Ventricular Tachycardia, it still takes the heart time to start producing adequate contractions. After the 2 minutes, then a pulse/rhythm check should occur.
- **Defibrillation** essential stops all electrical activity in the heart, we hope by doing so, the hearts normal electrical pathways take over and the patient resumes normal sinus rhythm.
  - Early defibrillation for ventricular fibrillation and pulseless ventricular tachycardia is key. The longer a patient has been in these rhythms, the less likely they are to respond to being shocked. Therefore, it is ideal to defibrillate as soon as possible.
- **Cardioversion** provides a reset. The heart is vulnerable during repolarization (T wave on an ecg) to energy. If you accidentally deliver the cardioversion shock on the T wave, it could trigger ventricular fibrillation. To avoid this risk, cardioversion should always be synchronized to the R wave (Always sync to the R wave in cardioversion).
- **Key in mind: Is the patient stable or unstable?** This will determine how aggressive and rapid treatments should be.

Treatment of Ventricular Fibrillation:

- CPR
- Early Defibrillation (200 J)
- Epinephrine 1mg Q3-5 minutes
- Amiodarone 300mg then 150mg
- Reversible Causes: H's and T's

Ventricular Fibrillation

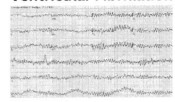

JerSISO, CC BY-SA 3.0 -https://creativecommons.org/licenses/by-sa/3.0-, via Wikimedia Commons

Treatment of Ventricular Tachycardia Without a Pulse:

- CPR
- Early Defibrillation (200J)
- Epinephrine 1mg Q3-5 minutes
- Amiodarone 300mg then 150mg
- Magnesium 2g if polymorphic
- Reversible Causes: H's and T's

Ventricular Tachycardia

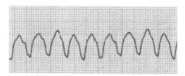

Gleniarson, Public domain, via Wikimedia Commons

Treatment of Ventricular Tachycardia with a Pulse:
- Synchronized Cardioversion (R Wave)
- Amiodarone Infusion Protocol (150mg over 10 minutes, followed by 1mg/min for 6 hours, then 0.5mg/min over 18 hours)
- Review H's and T's and potential triggers like any abnormal electrolytes

Ventricular Tachycardia

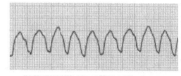

Gleniarson, Public domain, via Wikimedia Commons

Treatment of PEA and Asystole:
- CPR
- Epinephrine 1mg Q3-5 minutes
- Reversible Causes: H's and T's (Bicarb, Calcium, Fluids etc)

Pulseless Electrical Activity

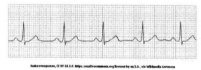

Andrewmeyerson, CC BY-SA 3.0 https://creativecommons.org/licenses by-sa3.0, via Wikimedia Commons

Treatment of SVT:
- Vagal Maneuvers
- Adenosine (6mg,12mg)
- Synchronized Cardioversion(Sync to R wave)

SVT

James Heilman, MD, CC BY-SA 3.0 <https://creativecommons.org/licenses/by-sa/3.0>, via Wikimedia Commons

Treatment of Symptomatic Bradycardia:

- Atropine 1mg Q3-5 minutes, max 3 mg
- Epinephrine Infusion
- Transcutaneous Pacing
- Identify possible triggers

Sinus Bradycardia

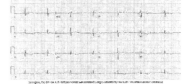

Treatment of 3rd Degree AV Block:

- Transcutaneous Pacing followed by Transvenous Pacing if available (Pacer will ultimately be inserted by cardiology)

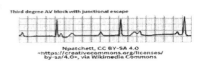

Treatment of Atrial Fibrillation with a Rapid Ventricular Response:

- IV fluids if no contraindication
- Metoprolol or Diltiazem IV (Followed by a PO dose for longer effect)
- Consider Amiodarone Infusion
- Consider synchronized cardioversion if new onset and no contraindications present

Atrial Fibrillation

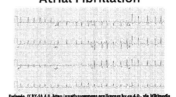

How to Defibrillate, Cardiovert and Pace

- Synced to the R wave with cardioversion
- When pacing, after electrical capture occurs, increase electrical current by 10-15% to ensure capture does not fail
- Ensure everyone is cleared prior to defibrillation and cardioversion
- After defibrillation, immediately resume CPR for another 2 minutes / 5 cycles

Defibrillation

The shockable rhythms are Ventricular fibrillation and Pulseless Ventricular tachycardia.

Ventricular Fibrillation

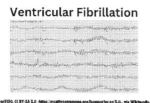

Ventricular Tachycardia

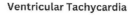
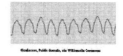

- Ensure pads are placed in an anterior posterior location, placing the heart between them. This allows the electrical current to pass directly through the heart.
- Turn the defibrillator on by turning the knob to "Defib"

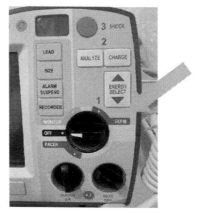

- Select the joules (amount of energy) for the defibrillation (You will be asking your provider this, however, it is typically between 120-

200J for biphasic)

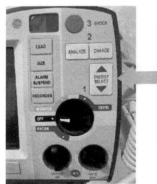 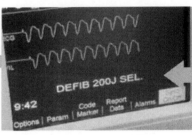

- Press Charge

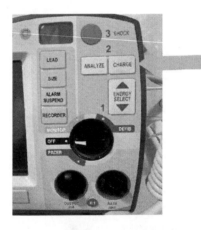

- Once charged, the orange button will light up. At that point, say "Everyone clear." Once everyone is cleared, press and hold the button to deliver the defibrillation.

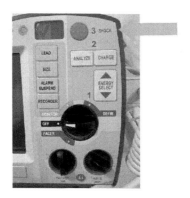

Cardioversion

Cardioversion will be used in rhythms such as SVT and ventricular tachycardia with a pulse to convert these abnormal rhythms back to normal sinus rhythm.

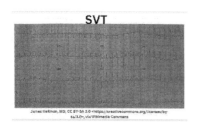

SVT

James Hellman, MD, CC BY-SA 3.0 <https://creativecommons.org/licenses/by-sa/3.0>, via Wikimedia Commons

Ventricular Tachycardia

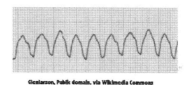

Glenlarson, Public domain, via Wikimedia Commons

- Ensure pads are placed in an anterior posterior location, placing the heart between them. This allows the electrical current to pass directly through the heart.
- Turn the defibrillator on by turning the knob to "Defib"

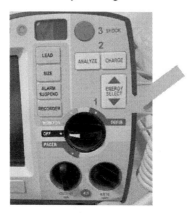

- Press the sync button (These will ensure the delivery of the electrical current occurs on the R wave)

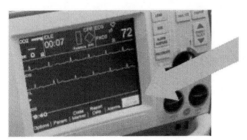 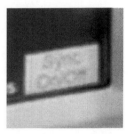

- Once synced, you should see markers/spikes/arrows above each R wave

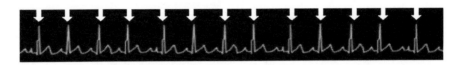

- Select the joules (amount of energy) for the cardioversion (You will be asking your provider this, however, it is typically between 100-200J for biphasic)

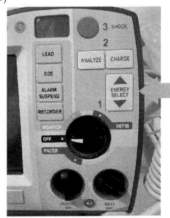

- Press Charge

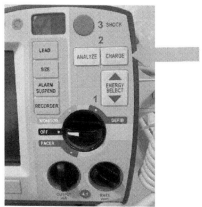

- Do one last check to ensure you are still synced by looking for those cardioversion markers above each R wave.

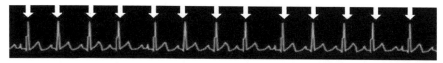

- Once charged, the orange button will light up. At that point, say "Everyone clear." Once everyone is cleared, press and hold the button to deliver the cardioversion.

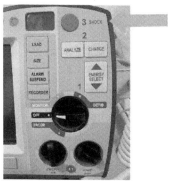

Pacing

Besides the pads being placed, for pacing, ensure the 3 Lead ecg from the monitor/defibrillator are also connected to the patient. The pads provide the electrical current to stimulate the heart, while with the 3 lead ecg, you will be able to see if there is electrical capture.

- Turn the knob to "pacer"

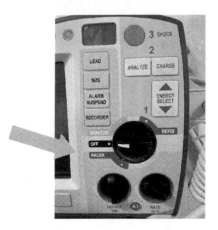

- Determine what the desired heart rate is (Ask your provider) and set it

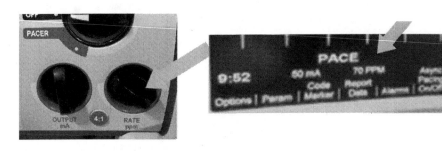

- Begin increasing the electrical output until there is electrical capture (electricity is causing a contraction)

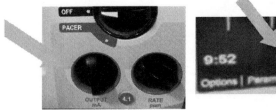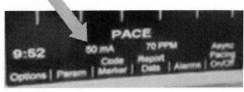

- Electrical capture is evident when there is a QRS following each pacer marker (as shown by the arrows)

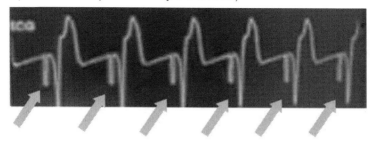

- After there is electrical capture, increase the electrical current by another 10-15% to ensure electrical capture does not fail. THEN, also manually check the heart rate to ensure a heart rate is produced (this is called mechanical capture).

ECG's

The ECG is a recording of the electrical activity of the heart. We can analyze the rhythm, assess for conduction issues and determine if there are signs of ischemia.

Normal Electrical Activity

The electrical impulse will start at the Sinoatrial (SA) node(in the right atria) and travel down the atria causing them to contract. It will then reach the atrioventricular (AV) node. The AV node holds the electrical signal for a brief moment to allow the atria to fully contract and the ventricles to fill with blood. Then the signal goes down the Bundle of HIS, to the right and left bundle branches and ultimately the purkinje fibers, causing the ventricles to contract.

ECG

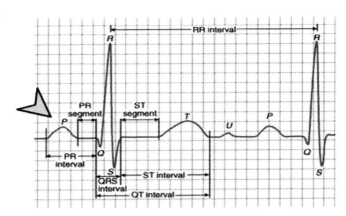

The ECG waveform goes as follows: P -> Q -> R ->S -T, then it repeats. It follows the conduction pathway of the heart.

- P Wave: represents atrial depolarization or atrial contraction. The P wave originates in the SinoAtrial node, which is why if there are P waves, it is called a "Sinus" rhythm.
- QRS Complex: represents ventricular depolarization or contraction. A normal QRS complex is less than 0.12 seconds. A widened QRS can signify significant issues like ventricular tachycardia, worsening hyperkalemia, a Bundle Branch Block, or even as a result of certain

44

medications/toxins. It can also be as a result of having a paced rhythm or from Premature Ventricular Contractions (PVCs')

- T Wave: represents ventricular repolarization or the ventricles relaxing and getting ready to contract again.
- PR Interval: From the beginning of the P wave to the beginning of the QRS complex. Helps assess how long it takes for the electrical signal to go from the atria to the ventricles. Normal duration is between 0.12 to 0.20 seconds. If it's prolonged, or longer than normal, it can mean that there is an issue with the AV node such as a heart block or ischemia that is affecting the SA or AV node.
- RR Interval: The time between the R waves of QRS complexes. Used to note whether the rhythm is regular if each R wave is the same length from each other and can quickly help us determine how fast the heart rate is by the length of the RR Interval. Varying RR intervals suggest an irregular rhythm, such as atrial fibrillation.
- QT Interval: From the beginning of the QRS complex to the end of the T wave. It shows how long it takes the ventricles to depolarize and repolarize. If the QT interval is long or becoming longer, we worry that the patient may go into a deadly arrhythmia like Torsades de Pointes. A baseline prolonged QT interval also prompts providers to avoid medications that have been known to cause arrhythmias and may cause providers to assess underlying electrolyte levels like magnesium (low levels may promote Torsades de Pointes).
- ST Segment: A key component of the ECG that helps assess for myocardial injury or ischemia. See below for more details.

<u>Rhythms to Recognize</u>

Normal Sinus Rhythm

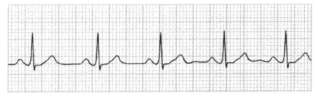

Andrewmeyerson, CC BY-SA 3.0 -https://creativecommons.org/licenses/by-sa/3.0-, via Wikimedia Commons

Ventricular Tachycardia

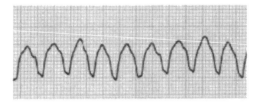

Glenlarson, Public domain, via Wikimedia Commons

Ventricular Fibrillation

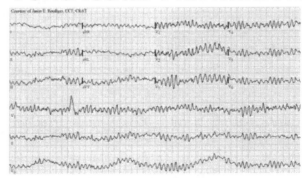

Jer5150, CC BY-SA 3.0 -https://creativecommons.org/licenses/by-sa/3.0-, via Wikimedia Commons

Atrial Fibrillation

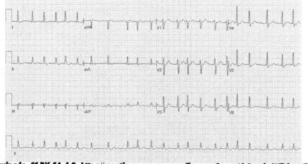

Pulseless Electrical Activity

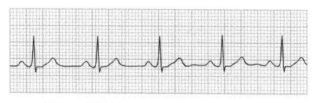

Sinus Tachycardia

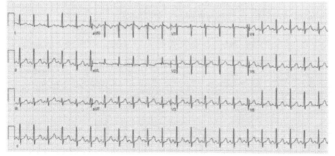

Sinus Bradycardia

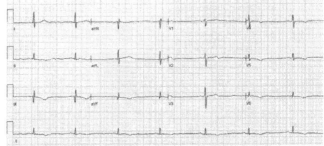

First degree AV block

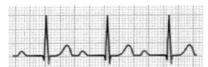

Second degree AV block (Mobitz I or Wenckebach)

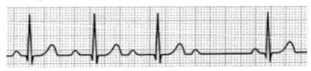

Second degree AV block (Mobitz II)

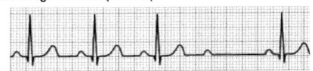

Second degree AV block (2:1 block)

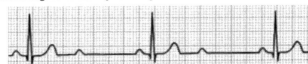

Third degree AV block with junctional escape

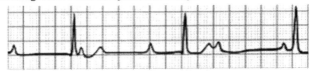

Remember that as a New ER nurse you should learn to recognize certain rhythms and signs of ischemia. The job of fully interpreting an ECG falls on the ER provider, and at times they don't even know so cardiology has to get involved, so be patient with yourself.

Interpreting the Basics of an ECG

So how should you go about it?

- **Is it sinus?**
  - Is there a P wave before every QRS? If there is, then it is sinus.
  - If not sinus, potential rhythms include Afib, Heart Blocks, Junctional, AFlutter, VT/VFIB
- **Is it regular?**
  - Is the RR interval the same throughout? Or are they different lengths from each other and therefore irregular?
  - If not regular, potential rhythms include Afib, Heart Blocks, Sinus Arrhythmia, VT/Vfib
- **What is the rate?**
  - Normal for adults is 60-100. Is the patient, brady tachy or normal?
  - You can use the 300 Method or 6 second method to quickly assess heart rate
  - If low, can include heart blocks and sinus bradycardia
  - If high, can include SVT, Aflutter, Afib, Sinus Tach, Vtac
- **Is the QRS normal? Or wide? Or progressive widening?**
  - If wide it can signal worsening Hyperkalemia or OD from a toxin, Bundle Branch Block, Ventricular Tachycardia or Ventricular Fibrillation
- **Signs of ischemia?**
  - ST changes(depression or elevation) in consecutive leads?
  - Inverted T waves?
- **Do I recognize the rhythm?**
  - You know what normal sinus rhythm looks like, does it look like it? If not, have someone with experience quickly assess it, especially in patients who are ill appearing.

Again, as a new ER nurse you don't have to be a pro, but you need to at least be able to recognize certain rhythms, when ischemia is occurring, and whether there are changes to the ECG so you can quickly get someone with more experience and qualifications (aka your provider) to read the ECG and make a care decision.

The more you practice the better you will be. Think of the answer and see what your provider went with and compare your answer and ask questions as to why. That way little by little you will get better. **If your organization offers an ECG course please take it!**

STEMI and Consecutive Leads

Now lets go over consecutive leads. Consecutive leads just mean part of the ecg that are looking at the same region of the heart.

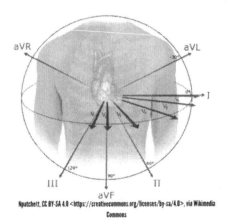

Npatchett, CC BY-SA 4.0 <https://creativecommons.org/licenses/by-sa/4.0>, via Wikimedia Commons

It's extremely useful to know about consecutive leads because if signs of ischemia are present, you can tell what part of the heart is being affected by which leads have the ischemia in.

I Lateral	aVR	V1 Septal	V4 Anterior
II Inferior	aVL Lateral	V2 Septal	V5 Lateral
III Inferior	aVF Inferior	V3 Anterior	V6 Lateral

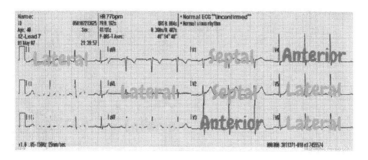

- **ST segment elevations in leads II, III, and aVF**
  - Indicates inferior MI with an occlusion of the Right Coronary Artery since it typically supplies blood supply to that section of the heart.
- **ST segment elevations in leads v5, v6, I, and aVL**
  - Indicates a lateral MI with an occlusion to the Left circumflex coronary artery since it commonly supplies that section of the heart.
- **ST segment elevation in V1-V4**
  - Indicates a septal anterior MI with an occlusion to the Left anterior descending coronary artery (LAD)

It's crucial to know this because when there are changes to consecutive leads, it is more likely that something is going on and it points directly to what part of the heart the issue is in. If the patient is having a STEMI and goes to the cath lab, the cardiologists will know exactly what vessel they have to go to and put a stent in.

Key Point: A quick point on electrolyte disturbances and ECG rhythms. **Do not forget to check the levels of electrolytes**. If your patient keeps going in and out of a deadly rhythm like ventricular tachycardia, how are the electrolytes? Could it be caused by a high or low potassium level? Or a magnesium disturbance? What about calcium and sodium?
The heart loves balance, especially when it comes to electrolytes. So when your patient keeps on having rhythm issues, don't forget to check the electrolytes.

Workup of Common Complaints

Providers will make a list of the possible diagnoses of the patient's chief complaint (the differential diagnoses) including the most life threatening conditions. The ER's job is to take care of emergencies so the providers will go down the list of the potential causes to ensure the life threatening and time sensitive issues are detected and treated. The goal is to rule out the out the deadly things first.

We as nurses are also on the lookout for these deadly conditions, especially in triage. We assess patients who present unstable so they can be prioritized and evaluated by a provider faster. For example, patients with unstable vital signs, altered level of consciousness, visible respiratory distress, pale mottled or cyanotic skin color, diaphoretic, vomiting and so forth.

The depth of the workup ordered will depend on how the patient presents, their vitals, the history and physical exam and risk factors such as age and known medical problems.

Our role as the ER Nurse is to carry out these orders proficiently and in a timely manner. We will administer medications, coordinate with radiology (Xray, Ct, US), and send off lab work. We will continually assess and monitor, communicating promptly when needed.

Chest Pain

Chest pain is a very common chief complaint in the ER. Among the deadly conditions of the differential diagnoses include Acute Coronary Syndromes (STEMI, NSTEMI, UNSTABLE ANGINA), CHF Exacerbation, Pulmonary Embolism, unstable ECG rhythms, pneumo's, dissections, valvular stenosis, pericarditis and asthma/copd exacerbations.
The workup can include an ECG, Labs, Chest X-rays, ultrasounds, and CT scans.
- ECG: Obtained within 10-15 minutes of the patient arriving as it can help identify signs of ischemia and ACS, as well as dangerous arrhythmias
- Labs: Can include Troponins, BNP, and a D-Dimer. A Basic Metabolic Panel (BMP) and a Complete Blood Count (CBC) is

usually obtained as well. Troponin helps identify heart muscle damage, the BNP helps with identifying heart failure, and D-Dimer can help with identifying Pulmonary Embolisms.

- Chest Xray: Helps look for pulmonary issues like pneumonia, pneumos and pleural effusions. Can also detect cardiomegaly.
- Echocardiogram: Helps assess how well the heart is pumping (Ejection Fraction), valves, and heart muscle issues.
- CT Scans: More detail of organ structures and vessels, for example if to rule out a Pulmonary Embolism.

Shortness of Breath

Among the deadly conditions of the differential diagnoses include Pneumo's, Pulmonary Embolisms, Asthma and COPD exacerbation, Pneumonia, CHF, Anemia, Anaphylaxis and ACS.
The workup can include an Chest X-rays, ECG, Labs, ultrasounds, and CT scans.

- Chest Xray: Helps look for pulmonary issues like pneumonia, pneumos, pulmonary edema and pleural effusions. Can also detect cardiomegaly.
- ECG: Obtained within 10-15 minutes of the patient arriving as it can help identify signs of ischemia and ACS, as well as dangerous arrhythmias
- Labs: D-Dimer, BNP, Troponins, ABG, CBC, BMP
  - ABG: Helps assess oxygenation, ventilation, and acid-base status
  - D-Dimer: Assess for Pulmonary Embolism. Often if positive (>500) a CT chest angiogram will be ordered to confirm PE
- CT: An Chest Angiogram may be ordered if pulmonary embolism is suspected. As well if more detail of organ structures is needed, for example, if something questionable was seen on the xray, the radiologist who read the chest xray will write "Recommend CT for further evaluation."
- Echocardiogram: Helps assess how well the heart is pumping (Ejection Fraction), valves, and heart muscle issues.

Abdominal Pain

Among the deadly conditions of the differential diagnoses include Aortic Dissection, GI Bleeding, perforated bowel, appendicitis, pancreatitis, cholecystitis, ectopic pregnancy and ruptured ovarian cyst. There are also countless other conditions that should be considered like UTIs, kidney stones, bowel obstructions and even gastritis.
The workup may include lab work, Ultrasounds, CT, and ECG.

- Labs: Pregnancy Test, Lipase and Amylase, LFT's, Urinalysis, CBC, BMP
    - Preg Test: Assess for pregnancy and to rule out related issues like ectopic pregnancy
    - Lipase Amylase: Evaluate pancreas
    - LFT's: Evaluate Liver and Gall Bladder
    - Urinalysis: Assess for UTI, DKA, kidney function
- Ultrasound: Assess for cholecystitis, appendicitis, ectopic pregnancies and intra abdominal issues
- CT: Will help provide more detailed information for possible pathologies in the abdomen
- ECG: To help rule out ACS with Atypical Presentations

Altered Level of Consciousness

Among the deadly conditions of the differential diagnoses include stroke(hemorrhagic and ischemic), hypoglycemia, hypertensive encephalopathy, hypoxia, hypercapnia, hepatic encephalopathy, electrolyte issues (hyponatremia), sepsis, seizures and toxic ingestions.
There is a useful mnemonic of issues to keep in mind with ALOC, AEIOU TIPS.

- A: Alcohol and Arrhythmias
- E: Electrolytes and Epilepsy
- I: Insulin
- O: Overdose and Oxygen
- U: Uremia
- T: Trauma and Temperature
- I: Infection
- P: Poison and Psych
- S: Stroke

The workup may include lab work, xray, CT, ECG and EEG.
- Labs

- o Point of Care Glucose: Assess for hypoglycemia or hyperglycemia
- o Urine Drug Screen and Serum Toxicology: Assess for OD of a substance
- o Troponin: Assess for ACS
- o CBC, BMP: Assess electrolytes, Infection, Kidney Function, Hgb
- o If indicated:
  - Ammonia: Liver Failure
  - CSF (Will need Lumbar Puncture): Infection in Spinal Fluid
  - Coagulation: Assess for bleeding disorders that increase risk of bleeding(Head bleeds)
  - VBG: Assess lactate level and approximate estimate of other values like CO_2
  - BNP: Assess for heart failure
- Chest Xray: Hypoxia can cause ALOC. A chest xray can help assess for pulmonary conditions contributing to the ALOC such as pneumonia, pulmonary edema, pneumothorax and so forth.
- ECG: Can help assess for issues that may be affecting perfusion such as arrhythmias and ACS
- CT: Help assess for abnormalities within the brain like brain bleeds and even tumors
- EEG: Can help assess for seizure

ALOC can have many causes and when patients also present unstable, the workup ordered can be rather extensive.

Syncope

Among the deadly conditions of the differential diagnoses include arrhythmias, heart failure, ACS, seizures, strokes, brain bleeds, hypoglycemia, hyperkalemia and toxins.
The workup can include lab work, ECG, Echocardiogram, chest xray, and CT.
- Labs
  - o Point of Care Glucose: Assess for hypoglycemia
  - o Troponin: Assess for ACS and heart muscle damage
  - o BNP: Assess for CHF if indicated

- CBC, BMP: Assess electrolytes, Infection, Kidney Function, Hgb
- Coags: Assess for bleeding disorders that increase risk of bleeding(Head bleeds)
- Urine Drug Screen and Serum Toxicology: Assess for OD of a substance
- ECG: Can help assess for issues that may be affecting perfusion such as arrhythmias and ACS
- Echocardiogram: If cardiac issues suspected. Helps assess how well the heart is pumping (Ejection Fraction), valves, and heart muscle issues.
- Chest Xray: Hypoxia and ventilation issues can potentially cause Syncope. A chest xray can help assess for pulmonary and cardiac conditions contributing to the syncope such as pneumonia, pulmonary edema, pneumothorax and cardiac enlargement.
- CT: A head Ct can help assess for intracranial issues like a head bleed that may have caused Syncope.

As you can see, there are many similarities in the workups. The depth of the workup ordered will depend on how the patient presents, chief complaint, their vitals, *the history and physical exam* and risk factors such as age and known medical problems.

Sepsis Workup

Sepsis is characterized by an infection and the body's unregulated reaction to the infection. What makes sepsis deadly is that it can eventually lead to multi-organ dysfunction and death.

The purpose of the sepsis workup is to locate the infection and figure out how sick the patient is. For example, is the patient already in organ dysfunction? Or are they still early on in the process. This is important to determine as it gives a sense of the patient's prognosis and determines how aggressive the team needs to be with interventions.

SIRS Criteria

Although I understand that guidelines are changing, many organizations still use SIRS criteria. As we know, sepsis is characterized by an infection, or a suspected infection and an unregulated immune response or again, in other words, SIRS. So when a patient comes into the ER, and you suspect the patient has an infection, you also need to go over the SIRS criteria to help assess whether the patient is septic and ultimately ensure they are placed as a priority. SIRS criteria has four components, 3 of which you can use in triage. They include a temperature greater than 100.4 F or less than 96.8F, a heart rate greater than 90, a respiratory rate greater than 20, and finally a wbc greater than 12,000 or less than 4,000.

Infection Symptoms

Symptoms that may indicate an infection can include fever, tachycardia, tachypnea, hypotension, fevers, chills and so forth. Again, these do not automatically mean that the patient has an infection, however, they can help guide the evaluation of the patient. For example, if the patient is febrile, tachycardic, has abdominal pain and green stools, it can help point the team in the right direction regarding the work up.

Key Point: Keep in mind that the most likely source of infection for septic patients are from the lungs, abdomen and urinary system.

Laboratory Studies for Infections/Sepsis

- **CBC**: The cbc with a differential will let us know the white count, what type of white blood cells are elevated and whether a shift is present.
- **CMP**: The CMP will let us assess for organ dysfunction and derangements as a result of the infection and the body's response.
- **Urinalysis**: The urinalysis will allow us to see if there is an infection in the urine and the urine culture will help us figure out which antibiotic is most effective.
- **Blood Cultures**: The blood cultures will help us detect whether bacteria is present in the bloodstream and figure out which antibiotic is most effective. The same principle applies if you obtain a culture from a different source, whether it is sputum, a wound or even from any type of tube or drain coming from the patient.
- **Lactate**: The lactate gives us an understanding of the patients perfusion status, whether tissues throughout the body are getting the oxygen and blood perfusion they need. Typically, the higher the lactate, the higher the mortality rate is. Its also useful to trend it, meaning you get a repeat lactate after initial interventions like fluids to gauge whether they are working.
- **Lumbar Puncture**: The LP will help us assess for an infection in the CSF if the patient is showing meningeal signs or even to rule out when the rest of the work up is inconclusive.
- **Other**: The team may also start ordering additional lab tests like inflammatory markers and a DIC panel. Inflammatory markers like **procalcitonin** help determine the level of inflammation throughout the body, the higher the level the higher the inflammation. The **DIC** panel will let us know if clotting factors are being consumed throughout the body, and signal whether they have to be replaced.

Source: The main thing I want you to remember is source control. Finding the source of the infection is crucial, especially when we keep trying everything and the patient is showing no signs of improvement. We need to address the source. The worst outcomes that I've seen is when we are unable to find the source. So is it coming from a skin infection somewhere?

From the foley? The central line? The pic line? The nephrostomy tube? The dialysis catheter? (Remember: Chest Abdomen Pelvis)

Radiology

The chest xray will help us figure out if the patient has pneumonia or any other condition that may be causing the patients symptoms. The same of the CT, itll help us find the source or perhaps help find the cause for the patients symptoms.

Treatment

- **Antibiotics**: As soon as the diagnosis is made, or even when there is a high suspicion of an infection being present, **antibiotics need to be administered.** Start off with **broad spectrum** then more targeted towards the potential source, then when the results of the cultures come back, the antibiotics will be specific towards the offending agent. From my understanding, the faster abx are given, the better the outcomes.
- **IV Fluids:** Fluids should be administered, especially when hypotensive, tachy and with a high lactate. Typically NS and LR are preferred. **Usually initially it is 30ml per kg in adults.** Remember to adjust the dosing when patients have congestive heart failure.
- **Vasopressors:** If fluids did not help with the hypotension, vasopressors will be considered. The first line vasopressor for sepsis is norepinephrine, then most likely vasopressin.
- **Supportive:** You will also be managing any derangements and abnormalities as a result of the sepsis such as electrolyte issues, organ dysfunction and so forth.
- **Other**: The team may consider **glucocorticoids** when the fluids and pressors did not help with improving perfusion as they are thought to help with adrenal insufficiency when the patient is very critically ill.

Sepsis and Nursing Tips

- Remember to keep in mind the SIRS criteria when triaging patients with a suspected source of infection.
- Obtain blood cultures prior to the antibiotics.
- Your facility may employ specific time bundles such as obtaining blood cultures, a lactate, giving fluids and abx in a certain time frame from patient arrival, so ensure you become familiar with your organization's protocols. These bundles are to ensure there is no delay in the treatment of septic patients.
- Remember that norepinephrine is the typically first line agent in sepsis, and that it can go peripherally initially. If you do use it peripherally ensure you place a large bore IV in the ac.
- **Closely monitor your patient to ensure interventions are working and if not, that you are timely communicating with the team.**

Common Conditions: Workup, Treatment, Nursing Tips

STEMI

- An ST Elevation myocardial infarction is full blockage or near full blockage of a coronary artery that occludes blood flow to that section of the heart. If left untreated, cells will begin to die off and it will eventually affect the heart muscle and how it contracts. The ST elevation will be seen in consecutive leads, pointing to which artery is occluded (see ECG section for details).
  - The patient can present with pressure like chest pain, shortness of breath, nausea, diaphoresis, paleness. The CP often radiates to the neck, jaw and arms.
  - Do keep in mind that a STEMI may also present differently in women and diabetic patients with symptoms such as epigastric pain, nausea and a feeling of impending doom. Often described as "Somethings just not right."
- Specifics of the Workup
  - ECG: Should be done within 10 minutes of patient arrival to the ER. The faster a stemi is caught, the faster reperfusion therapies occur and the more cells/muscle is saved.
  - Labs
    - Cardiac Enzymes: Troponin (Troponin will start to rise at hour 2) which is why ECG is very important to detect early
    - Baseline labs like CBC, BMP, Coags
  - These patients may also get a chest xray and bedside ultrasound by providers, BUT when a STEMI is identified, it should take priority unless there is a high suspicion of other causes.
- Treatment
  - Reperfusion Therapy is the Definite treatment
    - PCI or Percutaneous Coronary Intervention is preferred as it is more likely to be successful in opening the occluded artery and perfusing the heart. It also doesn't come with the bleeding risks associated with giving a thrombolytic.

- If PCI is not available or the nearest hospital with PCI capabilities is too far, a Thrombolytic will be administered to break the occlusion/clot up. This can be Tenecteplase or Alteplase.
    - A thrombolytic will break up the blockage, restoring blood flow. As the nurse you will need to closely monitor this patient for signs of serious bleeding such as a head bleed or GI bleeding (gum bleeding is not too concerning), plus continuously monitor vitals and ECG rhythm for any changes.
    - Contraindications for thrombolytics: Active Bleeding or Bleeding conditions like hemophilia, recent surgery or head bleed or trauma, uncontrolled hypertension among others
- Provide Oxygen: Keep SPO2 above 95%
- Medications
    - Aspirin: An antiplatelet, essentially helps by preventing the clot from getting bigger. For adults, the typical dose will be 324mg.
        - Ensure the patient is not allergic and there are no signs of acute bleeding.
        - If allergic, Plavix should be given. It is also an antiplatelet that helps prevent the clot from getting bigger.
    - Nitroglycerin: Helps dilate coronary arteries, which improves blood flow to ischemic area and helps oxygenate ischemic cells. As discussed it also helps with preload and afterload reduction, which decreases the workload on the heart, demanding less from it.
        - Contraindication: Do not administer nitroglycerin with Right Sided MI's, which can be evidenced by ST Segment elevation in inferior leads (II, III, AVF) (a right sided ecg should also be performed here). The right side of the heart fills passively, if you decrease preload, you are

decreasing the amount of blood returning to the heart, and as a result decreasing cardiac output because there is less blood to be pumped out.
- Also avoid if pt is on sildenafil.
- IV Fluids
  - If it is a right sided MI and the patient is hypotensive, IV fluids may be ordered to help increase preload.
- Heparin
  - One of the main reasons for getting heparin is if the patient is going for PCI, it will help prevent blood clot formation on the stent, helping keep it open.
  - Of course, the other is that it helps prevent the clot from getting bigger.

- Nursing
  - Be familiar with contraindications for thrombolytics and monitor closely for bleeding if thrombolytics are given.
  - Closely monitor ecg rhythm as the heart is irritable/ischemic and may suddenly go into Vfib,vtach or even into a block if the SA node is affected.
  - Be aware of reperfusion injury. Since there was no blood flow and perfusion to cells, acids and inflammation began to build up and when reperfusion occurs, these harmful substances are sent out to the body. Plus those ischemic cardiac cells underwent changes and now that oxygen and perfusion have returned, they can be further damaged as a result.

NSTEMI

- An Non-ST Elevation myocardial infarction is partial blockage of a coronary artery that decreases blood flow to that section of the heart. If left untreated, cells will begin to die off and it will eventually affect the heart muscle and how it contracts.

- The patient can present with pressure like chest pain, shortness of breath, nausea, diaphoresis, paleness. The CP often radiates to the neck, jaw and arms.
- Do keep in mind that a NSTEMI may also present differently in women and diabetic patients with symptoms such as epigastric pain, nausea and a feeling of impending doom. Often described as "Somethings just not right."
- Specifics of the Workup
  - ECG: Should be done within 10 minutes of patient arrival to the ER. It can detect signs of ischemia such as T wave inversions and ST segment depression
  - Labs
    - Cardiac Enzymes: Troponin (Troponin will start to rise at hour 2) which is why ECG is very important to detect early
    - Baseline labs like CBC, BMP, Coags
  - These patients will also get a chest xray and bedside ultrasound by providers. An if indicted, additional testing like CT cans, may be ordered.
- Treatment
  - Aspirin: An antiplatelet, essentially helps by preventing the clot from getting bigger. For adults, the typical dose will be 324mg.
    - Ensure the patient is not allergic and there are no signs of acute bleeding.
    - If allergic, Plavix should be given. It is also an antiplatelet that helps prevent the clot from getting bigger.
  - Provide Oxygen: Keep SPO2 above 95%
  - Analgesia: Morphine or Fentanyl
    - Give slowly, especially in elderly. Keep an eye on respiratory drive and if needed place on endtidal CO2. But if you give slowly, should have no serious side effects.
  - Nitroglycerin
    - Helps dilate coronary arteries, which improves blood flow to ischemic area and helps oxygenate ischemic cells. As discussed it also helps with

preload and afterload reduction, which decreases the workload on the heart, demanding less from it.

- o Heparin Bolus and Infusion
  - An anticoagulant that prevents the occlusion from getting worse, giving the body time to start breaking down the clot on its own. When on the heparin drip, you will repeat the ptt(might be all the coags at your facility) at a set amount of time, to ensure that the patient is at a therapeutic level of heparin, typically ranging between 60-90.(This changes a bit by institution so know yours).
    - Monitor your patients for signs of bleeding.
    - Before starting the heparin infusion, you will need a baseline hgb, hematocrit and coags, plus ensuring there are no signs of bleeding such as dark black stools prior to infusion. (You dont want to make bleeding worse, however, sometimes benefits vs risks play a role)

- Nursing
  - o You may be asking, well if there is a clot, why aren't we breaking it down with a thrombolytic? Since there is still blood flow and perfusion as the coronary artery is not fully blocked, the risk of severe/deadly bleeding with a thrombolytic is not worth the risk.
  - o Giving aspirin and starting a heparin infusion give the body time to start breaking down the partial occlusion.
    - HOWEVER, these patients will still most likely undergo a diagnostic angiogram in the cath lab and if needed, a stent will be placed there (or other treatments like CABG-based on what cardiology recommends).
    - ALSO, we will continue to closely monitor these patients, ensuring the ischemia and damage to the heart is not worsening, and if it is, it warrants the patient go to the cath lab faster and undergo PCI.
      - We monitor by repeating the ECG and troponins Q4H, Q6H, or Q8H or whatever

cardiology recommends. If the troponin starts to rise and there are more changes to the ECG, again, that is when PCI is indicated.
- We also closely monitor the patient for worsening signs and symptoms such as worsening or new chest pain, shortness of breath, diaphoresis, nausea or even new arrhythmias.
  - As the RN, you will carry out the interventions and closely monitor, promptly communicating with the team.

Congestive Heart Failure Exacerbation

- The heart is weak and or stiff, making it unable to pump blood effectively to meet the body's demands. As a result, there is fluid back up into the body. Fluid builds up in the lungs and rest of the body, particularly the lower extremities in the form of pitting edema.
  - The patient can present with shortness of breath, weakness, dizziness, peripherally edema and chest pain.
- Specifics of the WorkUp
  - ECG: identify arrhythmias and any ischemic changes.
  - Chest X-ray: assess for pulmonary edema and cardiomegaly.
  - Echocardiogram: assess cardiac structure and function, including ejection fraction
  - Brain natriuretic peptide (BNP): assess severity of CHF and confirm diagnoses
- Treatment
  - Oxygen, Monitor, IV
  - Nitroglycerin
    - A vasodilator that reduces preload and afterload. By decreasing the amount of blood returning to the heart (preload), the workload on the heart goes down. By decreasing systemic vascular resistance (afterload), there is less resistance to pump against, making it easier for the heart to pump

blood out. This combination of decreasing preload and afterload improves cardiac output.

- Also does dilate coronary arteries, increasing perfusion and oxygenation to heart muscle. This is why it is used for angina.
  - Also avoid if pt is on sildenafil.
- o Furosemide (Lasix)
  - A diuretic. Through diuresis, preload is decreased because there is less blood volume returning back to the heart, further decreasing the workload of the heart. (Diuresis is the key with CHF because getting fluid out is what will mainly treat the patient)
- o Bipap (Bilevel positive airway pressure)
  - By providing positive airway pressure during inspiration and exhalation, collapsed alveoli are opened and the pressure forces fluids out of the lungs. Making it easier to breathe and oxygenate.
- o Reverse cause of exacerbation if known such as an arrhythmia, anemia, acs, drugs(cocaine, meth) etc
- Nursing: Be proactive with assisting your patient to urinate after lasix(Urinal, Bedside commode, purewick) since that is how they will get better and strict I/Os
  - o For IV placement, hold pressure on site until edema subsides enough for veins to be palpated and IV placed, use a longer catheter

Hypertensive Emergency

- To qualify as a hypertensive emergency there have to be signs of end organ damage. End organ damage would be exhibited on the workup and physical assessment. Are there ECG changes, renal or heart injury in the labs? Is the patient actively experiencing chest pain, sob, dizziness, headaches, nausea?
  - o There will most likely be a cause for the hypertensive emergency and it must be addressed. Issues such as medication non compliance, renal disease, heart failure, drug use or uncontrolled hypertension may be a cause.
- Specifics of the Workup (aimed at identifying causes and *severity of end organ damage*)

- Labs:
  - BMP: Assessing Electrolytes and ensuring nothing is missed
  - CBC: Abnormalities in the CBC can help guide towards more uncommon causes
  - Kidney Function: Creatinine, GFR, BUN (Assess for kidney damage)
  - Cardiac Enzymes: Troponin and BNP (Assessing for damage or strain on heart muscle)
  - Urinalysis: Assessing for protein or blood in urine (kidney damage)
- Chest X-ray: assess for pulmonary edema and cardiomegaly
- ECG: identify arrhythmias and any ischemic changes.
- CT: When indicated based on symptoms and physical, for example, a head CT for a hypertensive patient with neurological deficits to rule out intracranial issues like a brain bleed
- Treatment
  - In a true hypertensive emergency, the MAP (Mean Arterial Pressure) should be lowered by no more than 20% in the first two hours. End organ damage was occurring as a result of the BP being too high, you do not want to further contribute to the damage through hypoperfusion.
    - Of course, there are times when the BP should be rapidly lowered such as with brain bleeds.
  - Medications
    - The medication used to the lower the bp will depend on the patient and cause.
    - Slow IV Push Medications
      - Labetalol
        - A beta blocker used to rapidly lower BP as a slow IV Push over 2 minutes. Typical dosing in adults may range from 10-20 mg. May repeat dosing.
        - It will lower the BP while having minimal effects on cardiac output.

- Onset is within 5 minutes and can last up to 4 hours.
- Considerations
  - It is a beta blocker. If the heart rate is less than 60, or even on the lower side nearing 60, a different agent should be used so the heart rate does not drop, causing other issues.
  - While actively giving, set BP to take Q5 minutes to monitor effects closely.
  - Avoid in Asthma, COPD, heart blocks, and of course when the patient is bradycardic and or hypotensive.
  - Whenever giving an antihypertensive, have a very recent last set of vitals.
- Hydralazine
  - An arterial vasodilator that helps decrease BP. It can be unpredictable in how much it drops the bp, which is why it is often used second to Labetalol when an IVP med is needed. It may cause reflex tachycardia.
  - Adult dose is typically 10-20 mg per dose.
  - Onset is within 5-10 minutes and can last up to 2-4 hours.
  - Considerations
    - Whenever giving an antihypertensive, have a

very recent last set of vitals.
- While actively giving, set BP to take Q5 minutes to monitor effects closely.
- Infusion / Drip Medications
  - Nicardipine (Cardene)
    - A CCB that is frequently used as an infusion to bring BP when no special considerations are present.
    - Start Dose will often be 5mg/hr, titrate by 2.5 mg q 5-10 minutes, max of 15mg/hr.
    - Onset is within 5-10 minutes, duration 4-6 hours
    - ***While actively giving, set BP to take Q5 minutes to monitor effects closely.***
  - Nitroglycerin
    - Will primarily be used to lower BP as an infusion with congestive heart failure exacerbations when the BP is high as a result of volume overload.
    - Many times it will be used for a short period of time to stabilize the patient while in the ER, then will be discontinued prior to admission if pt is stable
    - Onset is within 2 minutes, lasts up to 10 minutes
    - Infusion start dose is typically 5mcg/min, titrate by 5-10mcg q 5 minutes, with a common max from 100-200mcg/min. (Please verify drips/infusions start rates, titrations, and max with your own facilities protocols)

- o *While actively giving, set BP to take Q5 minutes to monitor effects closely.*
  - • Also avoid if pt is on sildenafil.
- • Esmolol
  - o A cardioselective beta blocker. In the ER, *I have only used it for bringing the BP down in aortic dissections and for bringing the HR down in Afib RVR. Therefore, you will most likely not see it as an antihypertensive in other conditions.*
    - • It slows the HR down, therefore decreasing cardiac output and BP.
    - • Useful in Dissection because you don't just want to give a med that will only lower the BP, the body will response to this by increasing the HR and contractility, which will make the dissection worse. Esmolol helps with both bringing the HR down and BP.
  - o Fast on fast off. Onset within 1 minute and duration of only up to 9 minutes.
  - o Adult dosing with an infusion will typically require a loading dose followed by 50mcg/kg/min, titrating by 50mcg/kg/min q 5-10mins, max of 200mcg/kg/min (Please verify drips/infusions start rates,

titrations, and max with your own facilities protocols)
- Nursing: Recheck the Bp, ensure cuff is correct size and place appropriately. While actively giving BP meds, set your Bp q 5 minutes to closely monitor patient response. Give the meds time to work (don't keep stacking titrations without giving appropriate time to work).

Cardiac Tamponade

- Fluid accumulates around the heart, this compresses the heart preventing cardiac filling and effective contractions, ultimately leading to decreased cardiac output and shock.
    - Causes can include pericarditis, penetrating chest injuries and as a result of fluid overload such as a renal patient who has missed dialysis
    - Patients can present with shortness of breath, chest pain, distant heart sounds, jugular venous distention and signs of shock such as tachycardia, hypotension, dizziness, pale, diaphoretic and so forth. (These patients sometimes look like CHF patients)
- Specifics of the Workup
    - ECG: Can show ST changes throughout all leads, can also also have small low voltage QRS
    - Chest Xray: Findings can point the provider towards pericardial effusion and cardiac tamponade
    - Ultrasound: Bedside Ultrasound by your ER provider to help confirm diagnoses or formal echocardiogram if readily available
    - Labs: Can include Troponins and BNP
    - CT: A chest CT may be indicated if Chest xray and bedside ultrasound are not conclusive and more details are needed
- Treatment
    - Pericardiocentesis
        - Removes the fluid around the heart. Typically a needle is inserted to reach the pericardial sac with the guidance of ultrasound and the fluid is aspirated.

- o IV fluids: A bolus may be administered to help with preload and cardiac output while providers prepare for pericardiocentesis. This is only a temporary stabilizing treatment.
- o Vasopressors: Dobutamine may be used to help the heart contract better while providers prepare for pericardiocentesis. This is only a temporary stabilizing treatment. (I've also used norepinephrine in these situations).
- Nursing
  - o Your role as the ER nurse with the pericardiocentesis, besides ensuring consent and time out, will be to ensure your patients has support (its stressful feeling sick and docs telling you they are going to stab you in the chest), place them flat or slightly elevated, monitor vital signs closely and keep an eye out for arrhythmias(anytime you mess with the heart, it can go into an arrhythmia).

Aortic Dissection

- A tear happens in the wall of the aorta and blood is able to escape into this tear, separating the layers of the aorta wall. If left untreated, blood will continue to enter, leaving less and less blood to perfuse organs. It can also cause the aorta to rupture and the patient bleeds out internally.
  - o Causes include untreated hypertension and connective tissue disorders
  - o Patients will present with sharp or tearing chest or back pain, shortness of breath, paleness and overall signs of shock. Pt can also have a difference in BP from R to L arms. The decreased perfusion to organs can present as symptoms of that organ system for example decrease perfusion to brain may exhibit stroke like symptoms.
- Specifics of the Workup
  - o CT Angiography: Main diagnostic study to help providers diagnose an aortic dissection. Will tell us where it is and how severe.
  - o Labs: CBC, BMP, Renal Function, Cardiac Enzymes, D Dimer. Coags. Type and screen.

- Function tests like renal and cardiac are to eval extend of injury from hypoperfusion
- DDimer and coags will help with assessing clotting issues as a result of clotting factors and blood being used up by the dissection
- Type and Screen for surgery
    - ECG: Assess for any ischemic changes to the heart and or arrhythmias (Ive taken care of patients whos dissection was big enough to tamper with blood flow going to coronary arteries)
    - Chest xray: Findings can point the provider towards dissection
- Treatment
    - Surgery is the definite treatment for aortic dissection
    - Blood Pressure Control
        - To prevent dissection from worsening, GOAL is an SBP less than 120 (ideally around low 100's)
        - Esmolol is great because as described earlier it helps bring the heart rate and BP down.
            - If esmolol alone does not produce desired effects, may add Nicardipine (cardine) on top (I have had pts on both esmolol and cardene to keep Bp and HR at desired goal)
        - Pain medications
            - Pain increases HR and BP. I primarily have given Fentanyl doses in the past, but have also seen morphine be used.
- Nursing
    - Assess BP q 5 minutes on **Right Arm** to ensure close monitoring (ask for an A line). You will be giving several doses of pain meds so give slowly and monitor for respiratory depression (Place pt on Endtidal CO2). If a dissection is suspected early on, ensure you are communicating with radiology so your patient goes early for CT. These patients can tank pretty quickly, so ensure you are also communicating with Surgery team. Have at least two good working IV's.

Thoracic and Abdominal Aneurysms

- Aneurysms are a weakened part of the aorta wall that dilate and bulge, can ultimately rupture and the patient can internally bleed out.
- Thoracic Aneurysm: Can involve the ascending aorta, aortic arch and descending aorta.
    - Patients can present with tearing or sharp chest or back pain, difficulty breathing and horseness or difficulty swallowing depending on location.
        - If large enough it may also present as signs of shock.
        - There may be differences in blood pressure between L and R arm, depending on where the aneurysm is.
- Abdominal Aneurysms: Will involve the descending aorta
    - Patients can be asymptomatic or present with abdominal pain or back pain, a pulsating abdominal mass and or if large enough, may also present with signs of shock.
- Specifics of the Workup
    - CT Angiography: Help identify the presence, size and location
    - Ultrasound: Can also help identify the presence and size, however, CT is preferred
    - Labs: Aimed at identifying complications such as end organ damage and to obtain a baseline or identify comorbidities that may be present
        - CBC, BMP, Renal Function, Cardiac Enzymes, Coags, Type and Screen
    - ECG: Assess for any ischemic changes to the heart and or arrhythmias
    - Chest xray: as part of the initial workup prior to diagnoses being made
- Treatment
    - Surgical Repair or Stent/Graft Placement
    - Blood Pressure Control
        - Esmolol and if needed adding Nicardipine on top (Just as we discussed for dissection)
        - The goal is an sbp less than 120

- o Pain Control
  - Pain increases HR and BP. Will either give fentanyl or morphine (Just as we discussed for dissection)
- Nursing
  - o As with any other critical patient have 2 good working IV's, especially with these patients as they can tank fast if aorta ruptures. At that point blood products and a massive transfusion will be given(good IV's in these situations are life saving). Ensure you are coordinating with other healthcare teams to decide if the patient will be transferred or will be taking up for definite treatment (essentially help expedite it).

Pulmonary Embolisms

- A blood clot obstructs blood flow in the coronary arteries. The potential for rapid deterioration increases depending on the blood clots location and on its size. This blood clot will obstruct blood flow, leading to less oxygenated blood, less blood reaching the left ventricle and increases in pressure within the pulmonary arteries.
  - o As a result, patients can present hypoxic and Short of breath. Also tachycardic, with chest pain and with signs of low perfusion like dizziness, altered, diaphoretic. Ultimately, if the obstruction is severe and or worsening, hypotension and shock, with ultimate death as a result of poor cardiac output and low oxygenation.
  - o A very common cause is a DVT that broke off and ended up in the lungs. DVT occurs as a result of venous pooling (long flights or car rides) or hypercoagulable conditions like cancer, pregnancy or even recent surgery.
- Specifics of the workup
  - o D-Dimer: Forms when there is active breakdown of clots within the body, if elevated it does not confirm a PE, however, it further increases its likelihood, prompting the provider to perform additional testing
  - o CT Pulmonary Angiogram: Directly visualize pulmonary vascular to assess for blood clots, their location and size

- If the patient is severely allergic to contrast, a V/Q scan may be ordered if the patient is stable enough
  - ECG: Will most likely show sinus tachycardia and may show signs of right heart strain (blood backs up into the R side of the heart, placing strain)
  - Bedside Echocardiogram: your provider can look at the right ventricle looking for dilation and strain
  - To cover the general workup related to the patients presenting symptoms: a cbc, cmp, troponin will most likely also be ordered
- Treatment
  - If hypotensive, administration of fluids may be ordered. If hypotension persists, vasopressors may be ordered. If rapidly deteriorating, the blood clot needs to be rapidly broken down with a thrombolytic and or removed by interventially radiology.
  - Oxygen to help improve oxygenation and alleviate symptoms
    - High flow nasal cannula is preferred
  - If stable, Heparin Bolus and Infusion
    - An anticoagulant that prevents the occlusion from getting worse, giving the body time to start breaking down the clot on its own. When on the heparin drip, you will repeat the ptt(might be all the coags at your facility) at a set amount of time, to ensure that the patient is at a therapeutic level of heparin. Before starting the heparin infusion, you will need a baseline hgb, hematocrit and coags, plus ensuring there are no signs of bleeding such as dark black stools prior to infusion. (You dont want to make bleeding worse, however, sometimes benefits vs risks play a role)
  - If rapidly deteriorating, in shock or unstable, a thrombolytic should be administered to rapidly break down the clot.
- Nursing
  - Ensure you place a large bore IV for the CT Pulmonary Angiogram
  - Have multiple IV's for these patients, at least 2

- o Know your facilities heparin infusion protocol
- o Know the contraindications for thrombolytics
- o If heparin and or TNK were given, monitor closely for bleeding
- o You can assess if your patient will tolerate being flat for CT by simply lowering the head of the bed briefly. If they immediately becoming symptomatic, communicate with the team to form a plan

Asthma Exacerbation

- Characterized by inflammation, bronchoconstriction and mucus production that lead to patients having difficulty getting oxygen in and carbon dioxide out as the airways are inflamed, constricted and filled with mucus.
  - o Symptoms can include shortness of breath and wheezing, chest tightness and coughing. As it progresses, there will be little air movement (less wheezing), unable to speak, cyanotic, and increasing altered as they go into respiratory failure if nothing is done.
- Specifics of the workup
  - o The diagnosis of asthma is typically done from the history and physical examination, not labs or radiology. However, the general workup will still most likely be ordered to help rule out other issues and or possibly help identify causes/triggers
  - o Chest Xray, CBC, BMP, Bedside Ultrasound
- Treatment
  - o Oxygen: Alleviates hypoxia
  - o Albuterol and Ipratropium
    - Albuterol is a short acting beta agonists that helps relax bronchial smooth muscle, resulting in improved airflow from bronchodilation
    - Ipratropium Bromide is also typically administered with albuterol as it also helps with bronchodilation, further alleviating bronchospasm

- o Corticosteroids are given to help decrease the inflammation and edema present in the airways, further improving airflow
- o Magnesium: Also promotes bronchodilation by helping relax bronchial smooth muscle
- o Noninvasive Ventilation (Cpap/Bipap) helps improve ventilation and oxygenation through the constant positive airway pressure provided, helping alleviate hypoxia and hypercapnia.
- Nursing
  - o Learn to work closely with the respiratory therapists
  - o If you are working in a small ER, learn how to give a breathing treatment (albuterol/ipratropium)
  - o Closely monitor and promptly communicate with the team
    - Listen to the lungs, ensuring there is improve in air flow
    - If you do not hear much and the patient is in obvious distress, it means there is no movement of air as a result of the inflammation, bronchoconstriction and mucus

Pneumo/Hemothorax

- A pneumothorax is air in the pleural space while a hemothorax is blood. These can collapse the lung or impede it, ultimately affecting ventilation and gas exchange (hypoxia and hypercapnia). As they worsen, both will compress surrounding structures including the vena cava and heart, leading to decreased cardiac output. With hemothorax, if the bleeding is severe into the pleural space, blood loss will further cause hemodynamic instability. Tracheal deviation is a late sign.
  - o These patients will present with absent breath sounds on one side, shortness of breath, hypoxic, tachypnea, tachycardia and if severe, will start showing additional signs of shock like hypotension, paleness and ALOC.
- Specifics of the workup
  - o The physical examination is a very good indicator, specifically if there are absent breath sounds on one side.

- Chest Xray: For a hemothorax, there would be no lung markings on the affected side while with a hemothorax, there would be opacity/whiter on the affected side.
- Bedside Ultrasound by ER provider: Can visualize the lung and or fluid collection
- If the findings of the above are inconclusive, additional testing like a CT chest may be necessary for more detailed images. However, when severe enough, which prompt immediate treatment in the ER, they will be easily seen on a chest xray by your provider.
  - Hemothorax are commonly caused by trauma and these patients may receive a variety of CT scans to also assess for other injuries

- Treatments
  - Pneumothorax
    - A tension pneumothorax(severe version) will require immediate needle decompression to quickly allow air to escape the chest cavity, stabilizing the patient by decreasing the pressure on the lungs, heart and surrounding structures.
      - A chest tube will still be necessary to help restore the pressures within the pleural space. This will help the lung fully reexpand and eventually fully heal.
    - If the pneumothorax is small and not causing any instability, the patient may simply be placed on oxygen and monitored.
  - Hemothorax
    - A tension hemothorax (severe version) will require a chest tube to properly drain the blood from the pleural space.
      - If needed, to help with hypotension and hypoperfusion as a result of the blood loss, blood may be administered. A small fluid bolus may also be initially given.
      - If after chest tube placement, bleeding is ongoing, the patient may need to go to surgery to locate and control the source of the bleeding.

- o Oxygen Administration
    - ▪ I commonly place my patients on a nonrebreather initially until stabilized
- Nursing
    - o Ensure chest tube drainage device is placed somewhere where it will not get accidentally damaged or pulled
        - ▪ If accidentally pulled, place petroleum gauze or xeroform over it, ideally on exhale
        - ▪ Immediately call the team and let them know (It happens.. Learn from it and be more careful next time)
    - o Monitor for continued bleeding with hemothorax on the chest tube drainage. If the output begins to increase rapidly with more than 200ml per hour, or the color suddenly changes to bright red, notify the team
    - o Ensure supplies are ready for chest tube placement include chest tube, suction, drainage system, antiseptic, sterile gloves, gown and so forth.
    - o Ensure patient gets pain medications (or at least ensure a local anesthetic is used)
    - o Be proactive with calling xray after the chest tube is placed. The new chest xray will verify correct placement

Pneumonia

- An infection of the lungs. When it occurs in susceptible populations like the elderly or immunocompromised, it can lead to sepsis, respiratory failure, shock and death if left untreated.
    - o The inflammation can damage alveoli, leading to increased permeability that allows substances (fluids, proteins, wbcs) to accumulate in lung tissue. This leads to impaired gas exchange which may lead to hypoxia and CO_2 retention. As this progresses, worsening respiratory failure and septic shock can occur.
    - o These patients will present with signs of an infection such as fever, chills, tachycardia and fatigue. For pneumonia specifically, symptoms can include cough, sob, chest pain upon breathing.
- Specifics of the workup

- o Chest Xray: Helps identify presence of pna
- o Labs
  - CBC: assess level of wbc's and if with differential, can see type of white blood cells (whether mature or immature wbc's) or whether a viral etiology is more likely
  - BMP (Chemistry): helps assess for any abnormalities with electrolytes, kidney function and overall imbalances
  - ABG/VBG/Lactate: Help assess oxygenation, ventilation, acid base and perfusion status
    - If the patient is critical, an ABG is preferred over a VBG to obtain accurate values. Otherwise, VBGs may be used as they are easier to obtain and less painful for patients. But anytime, oxygenation and ventilation need to be accurately assessed, an ABG is preferred for its more accurate values.
  - Blood Cultures and Sputum Culture: help identify bacteria causing infection and help choose appropriate Antibiotic
  - CT Chest: If chest xray shows anything inconclusive, a chest ct may be ordered to obtain more detailed images. It can help assess for an abscess or pus collection.
- Treatment
  - o Oxygen administration to assist with treating hypoxia
  - o Fluid Administration when signs of sepsis are present such as tachycardia and hypotension. The adult initial resuscitation is 30ml/kg. Typically, normal saline is used.
    - If needed, for hypotension and shock, vasopressors should be used.
  - o Antibiotics. Obtain blood cultures first, then broad spectrum antibiotics immediately after. This will treat the infection present. Blood cultures are important so we can figure out which antibiotic the organism is more susceptible to.
  - o If viral source, the appropriate antiviral may be ordered.

- Supported care such as pain management and correction of any abnormalities that may arise from the derangement of septic shock if present.
- Nursing
  - Ensure timely and rapid administration of antibiotics once ordered. The earlier the better patient outcomes tend to be.
    - Do your best to obtain blood cultures prior.
  - Be aware of your facilities sepsis bundle and what it encompasses. It will most likely prioritize antibiotic and fluid resuscitation within a timeframe of suspicion.
  - Ensure patient comfort including appropriate pain management and antipyretics when needed.
  - Continuously monitor respiratory status to ensure improvement, and if worsening, promptly communicate with the team.
  - When elderly or immunocompromised patients come into the ER, be mindful of the main sources when severe infection can occur. These are the chest, abdomen and pelvis.

Intracranial Hemorrhage

- Bleeding occurs within the skull, either within the brain or in its surrounding structures. The blood places pressure on surrounding structures and increases ICP(Intracerebral Pressure). The increase in pressure irritates and reduces perfusion to the brain. If the bleeding is severe and ongoing, it places so much pressure on the brain that it can herniate (pops out of where its supposed to be) and critically reduces perfusion.
  - Causes can include head trauma, ruptured aneurysms, hypertension and use of anticoagulants.
  - These patients can present with severe sudden headaches, altered or comatose, nauseas and vomiting, seizing (the blood and pressure irritate the brain), and with other neurological deficits such as weakness, numbness, coordination and vision issues.

- There are different types of brain bleeds including Epidural, Subdural, Subarachnoid, and intracerebral hemorrhages. Epidural bleeding is from an artery (so it may continue expanding and be rapid onset). A subdural bleed is from a vein, so it may be slow in onset. A subarachnoid bleed is typically from a ruptured aneurysm.
- Specifics of the workup
  - Point of care glucose: to rule out hypoglycemia as cause of symptoms
  - Head CT: This is the key workup as providers are able to clearly visualize the location and size of the bleeding. A non-contrast head CT will also help assess for other conditions that may cause similar symptoms and if nothing is found, it may prompt the providers to order additional testing such as a perfusion study
  - Coagulation: To help assess coagulopathies, and if present, providing reversal agents like Kcentra or FFP depending on cause. Reversing is important to prevent ongoing bleeding.
  - CBC: Ensure no abnormalities with platelets, or other issues like anemia or increased WBCs
  - BMP (Chemistry): helps assess for any abnormalities with electrolytes, kidney function and overall imbalances
- Treatment
  - ABCs: If the patient is comatose or a rapidly decreasing GCS, intubation should be considered for airway protection
  - Blood Pressure Control: Goal is to maintain an SBP less than 140
    - Nicardipine Drip
    - Labetalol Slow IV Push
  - Seizure Prophylaxis: Keppra (Levetiracetam)
  - Anticoagulant Reversal
    - Depending on agent being reversed: Vitamin K, FFP, Kcentra, Platelets, Protamine Sulfate
  - If impending herniation
    - Mannitol and Hypertonic Saline: helps draw fluid out of brain tissue, creating more space within the skull to lower ICP. Hypertonic saline is most commonly used.

- o Surgical Intervention
  - Depending on the type of bleed, neurosurgery can drill a hole and evacuate the bleed/hematoma. Or even remove an entire section of the skull to alleviate the increase in pressure within the skull
- Nursing
  - o If neurosurgery will be placing a drain, have the drainage device ready
    - Be prepared to go to CT immediately after to verify placement of drain
    - Know how to zero and level the device, an ICP above 20 is critical, if up trending, also notify the team
  - o Cerebral Perfusion Pressure(CPP): MAP - ICP. CPP should be remain above 60. If not, communicate with the team to figure out interventions.
    - To obtain ICP, neurosurgery will need to insert an intraventricular device (IVD)
  - o A repeat head CT will be done 6 hours after to assess whether the bleed has gotten bigger or if it stayed the same
  - o Closely monitor blood pressure and titrate nicardipine as directed. Notify the team if nicardipine is maxed out and BP is still not under control
  - o Neuro assessments Q1 hour and or more frequent if needed

Seizures

- Uncontrolled/abnormal electrical activity within the brain that typically involves loss of consciousness and jerking like movements. If prolonged seizure activity or multiple seizures in a short amount of time, damage to the brain can occur as a result of changes in blood flow and oxygenation combined with an increased metabolic demand.
  - o There are different types of seizures and each can present differently. However, in the ER we will focus on seizures that present with jerking like movements, alterations in mentation and confusion. Patients also very commonly present with oral(tongue) trauma from accidentally biting it,

and incontinence. During the seizure, patients will become tachycardic, so keep an eye on the cardiac monitor for sudden increases in heart rate as your patient could be having a seizure.
- o Causes can include underlying seizure disorders where the patient has not been taking their medications or there has been a change in them, hypoglycemia, hyponatremia, delirium tremens, brain bleeds, toxins and even brain infections.
- Specifics of the workup
  - o Point of Care Glucose Check: Rule out hypoglycemia as the cause
  - o BMP (Chemistry): Assess electrolytes, such as sodium as hyponatremia can cause seizures. Helps also assess any other abnormalities present
  - o CBC: Help determine if an infection is present if the wbcs are high (meningitis etc). I've also had patients in the past who had an underlying seizure disorder and seized as a result of their hgb being low
  - o Urine Tox Screen: Assess for drugs that are uppers and promote seizure activity in those susceptible, drugs like cocaine and meth
  - o Heat CT: Especially useful in first time sz, to rule out a brain pathology like a tumor, to help rule out brain bleeds, brain abscesses and other conditions
  - o EEG: Helps assess electrical abnormalities of the brain (like an ecg for the heart this is for the brain). Useful to determine if patient is continuously seizing, prompting more aggressive treatment and management
  - o Lumbar Puncture: If rest of workup inconclusive, an LP may be useful for ruling out conditions like meningitis
- Treatment
  - o Active Seizure: Turn the patient onto their side and place oxygen. Notify your provider and prepare to give medications to help stop the seizure
  - o Medications
    - First line medications are benzodiazepines. Intramuscular Midazolam if not IV access is present. Intravenous Lorazepam if IV is present. IV

Lorazepam is preferred as it will start to work fast and will have long lasting anti seizure effects. However, if an IV is not present, IM Midazolam works faster to control a Sz compared to IM Lorazepam.

- Second line medications can include levetiracetam, phenytoin and valproic acid. Most commonly, levetiracetam (keppra) is used. It is given IV.
  - By this point, after giving a benzo and keppra, most seizures stop.
- If the seizure is ongoing or the patient continues to have additional seizures repeated, intubation may be considered in order to provider more aggressive treatment which can include medications like infusions of propofol and midazolam, as they both have antiseizure properties. Phenobarbital may also be used.

o Treat the underlying cause!
  - If its as a result of hypoglycemia, give dextrose. If its hyponatremia, give some hypertonic saline. If its because the patient has not been taking their meds, give a loading dose. If its a brain bleed, proceed down that pathway. If an infection, give antibiotics. Again, the important thing will be to treat the underlying cause of the sz, so keep that in mind while you are doing the interventions.

- Nursing
  o If the patient came in confused (post ictal) continuously monitor and chart their progress.
  o Have seizure precautions in place. Padded side rails, gurney in lowest position, patient within nursing station view if possible.
  o Ask your provider ahead of time if the patient has another seizure, what medication and dose would they like to be administered.
  o Memorize the questions to ask for seizures (review guide to questioning)

Ischemic Stroke

- A blood clot blocks blood flow to a region of the brain and within minutes brain tissue can begin to die due to lack of oxygen, glucose and other substances. It is crucial to rapidly restore blood flow to prevent permanent brain damage
  - Symptoms can vary depending on the location of obstruction and how much of the brain is affected. Common symptoms will include unilateral numbness or weakness, facial droop, slurring or difficulty understanding speech, coordination issues, headaches and dizziness.
- Specifics of the workup
  - The physical examination is the main key to recognizing a stroke.
  - Poc Glucose: to rule out hypoglycemia as the cause
  - Head CT: To rule out other causes of the patients symptoms, especially to rule out an intracranial hemorrhage. The head noncon CT needs to happen prior to the rest of radiological studies and any other interventions.
  - CT angiography and perfusion study: Using contrast, will be able to visualize arteries to locate where the occlusion is occurring
  - MRI: Will be useful to clearly see where there is damage in the brain. MRI's are specifically useful with wake up strokes, so we can assess whether there is any tissue left to be saved. If the tissue has died off and we give a thrombolytic, we can cause a brain bleed through the dead tissue
  - Coagulation Studies: To assess for coagulopathies that may be a contraindication to thrombolytics
  - CBC and BMP: To assess for any other abnormalities that may be present
- Treatment
  - Thrombolytic administration within 4.5 hours of symptom onset and after head CT to rule out brain bleed
    - Know absolute contraindications and relative contraindications

- - Know what your facility uses whether TNK or TPA as they have different protocols for administration.
  - Endovascular Thrombectomy
    - Interventional radiology will remove blood clot using a catheter/wire typically inserting through the groin
    - Used when the blood clot is big as a thrombolytic may not be enough to fully break it down.
    - Typically very useful within 4-6 hours, but may be done up to 24 hours if indicated based on the imaging
  - If patient does not meet criteria for Thrombolytic therapy or thrombectomy
    - Permissive Hypertension: Allow the bp to go as high as 220/120 to help maintain perfusion to the area, hoping no additional brain tissue dies from lack of perfusion
    - Physical Therapy, Occupational Therapy and Speech Therapy
    - Prevent further strokes
- Nursing
  - Memorize the symptoms of a stroke and activate the stroke protocol when necessary
  - Know the contraindications of thrombolytics
  - Thrombolytics should be administered with 4.5 hours of symptom onset
  - Know when the last seen normal was
  - Check a poc glucose first to rule out hypoglycemia
  - Place the IV in the AC or upper Forearm. 18 G is ideal for angiogram and perfusion study. At least two IV's prior to thrombolytic, the patient should not have anything invasive after due to risk of bleeding
  - Obtain a set of vitals early on as hypertension (above 180/110) is a contraindication for thrombolytics. An antihypertensive would need to be given such as Labetolol SIVP
  - Obtain an accurate patient weight as both TNK and TPA are weight based medications

- If you gave a thrombolytic, that patient would become a 1:1 patient
    - The risk for significant and deadly bleeding is always present. Closely monitor your patient and if they have a sudden decrease in mentation or change in status, notify your team. I've had several of my patients in the past develop an intracranial hemorrhage after thrombolytic administration

Gastrointestinal Bleeding

- GI bleeds refer to bleeding anywhere along the GI tract from mouth to anus. Its typically separated as upper GI bleeding (esophagus, stomach, duodenum) and Lower GI bleeding(rest of small intestine, colon, rectum and anus). Can be deadly when there are great amounts of blood lost, especially when it occurs rapidly.
    - If the bleeding is severe, signs of hemorrhagic shock may be present such as paleness, hypotension, tachycardia, aloc, or dizziness. As well as abdominal pain/discomfort and nausea.
        - Upper GI Bleed: Bright red emesis or coffee ground emesis, Black Stools
        - Lower GI Bleed: Bright red stool
    - Causes can include peptic ulcers, esophageal varices, gastritis, cancer, diverticulosis and hemorrhoids.
        - Chronic alcohol use is associated with gastritis and liver issues, which make patients more prone to GI bleeding
        - Chronic NSAID use also places patient at an increased risk of GI bleeding
- Specifics of the workup
    - Labs
        - CBC: Assess hgb, hematocrit and platelets
        - BMP: Assess electrolytes and kidney function to determine if injury is occur to other organ systems from the GI bleeding (lack of perfusion)
            - Liver function tests: to assess the Liver as it plays a role in clotting
        - Coagulation: Assess Pt, ptt, INR

91

- - Type and CrossMatch: To give the patient blood products if needed (If your provider forgets to order, remind them)
    - Lactate: helps assess perfusion status and we can trend to verify treatments are having a positive effect
  - Guaiac Testing: Directly assess for blood in stool
  - CT Angiography: Help determine where in the GI tract bleeding is occuring
  - Esophagogastroduodenoscopy (EGD): Through a long scope/catheter that has a camera attached, the GI provider can directly visualize the Upper GI tract and if source of bleeding is located, can treat with banding, clipping or cauterization
- Treatment: How aggressive the treatment will depend on whether the patient is stable or unstable
  - Blood Products including PRB's, FFP and Platelets
    - If bleeding is not severe, a fluid bolus can be given
  - If severe enough, A Massive Transfusion with high numbers of blood products through a rapid transfuser (can deliver entire units of bleed within minutes)
  - Medications
    - Proton Pump Inhibitor: helps decrease acid reduction to promote healing
    - Octreotide: Used primarily when variceal bleeding is suspected as it helps reduce portal hypertension, which helps decrease the amount of bleeding. This effect is also useful post treatment/fixing to help prevent rebleeding. You will typically give a bolus/push then start an infusion at a set rate.
    - Antibiotics: Will be given to prevent infections such as SPB(Spontaneous Bacterial Peritonitis)
  - Blakemore or Minnesota Tube: Places pressure on the bleeding site (especially esophageal varices). This is a stabilizing measure, giving the team time to initiate other interventions.
  - EGD: Banding, Clipping

- o Embolization by Interventional Radiology: Essentially, cutting blood supply to bleeding area
  - o Surgical Repair
- Nursing
  - o Place additional priority on unstable GI bleeds as they can rapidly deteriorate and Code
  - o Know how to use your organizations rapid blood transfusion and if Massive Transfusion Protocol is activated, discuss with your provider unless protocol is clearly detailed, how many Units of RBCs vs platelets vs FFP (what ratio do they want)
  - o Multiple IV's as different medications and interventions will be implemented. If the patient requires a massive transfusion, a large bore IV is ideal for rapid administration of blood

Hypoglycemia

- A low blood glucose level. Technically less than 70, however, symptoms typically start once levels start dropping below 60. The body as a whole will suffer from low glucose levels, however, the brain and heart are most notable. If hypoglycemia is severe and prolonged, permanent brain damage will occur. The heart will also suffer from hypoglycemia as the body will be in a stress response, prompting the heart to beat faster and faster while having little glucose for energy. This demand will eventually lead to arrhythmias and eventual cardiac arrest.
  - o Patients can present with shakiness/tremors, pale and sweaty, tachycardic, confused/altered. As it progresses, worsening confusion, loss of consciousness, seizures and eventually heart issues and death if left untreated.
  - o Causes are most commonly from insulin issues and diabetic medications, whether taking too much insulin or their regular Sulfonylureas or even not eating when they are supposed to.
    - Other very important causes you need to be aware of include hypoglycemia as a result of sepsis, liver failure and hypothermia. I want to highlight sepsis specifically. Check a point of care glucose with

critical septic patients regularly. There's been plenty of times when these patients were relatively stable and suddenly started decompensating and no one could figure out why until a more seasoned nurse said "Has anyone checked the sugar?"

- Specifics of the workup
  - Poc Glucose Testing: To assess glucose level
  - Health and History Assessment/Questioning: Crucial in identifying use of insulins and diabetic medications, their last use, dose and if patient ate. You should also be inquiring about any potential illness(infectious sources) and whether the patient has been binge drinking alcohol (when this happens patients tend not to eat).
  - The basic workup will also be done to help assess overall patient status including a CBC and BMP.
    - If suspected, cortisol levels for adrenal issues. Liver Function as the liver also plays a role in glucose levels and other very specific tests (not common).
  - These patients, as they are often confused/altered, will also get the altered workup to ensure nothing is missed. Mainly a head CT to ensure no intracerebral issues.
- Treatment
  - If the patient is awake, alert, protecting their airway and able to swallow, eating is the first line. Typically in the ER, we'll have them drink juice (some nurses add an extra sugar packet) then provide them with a meal.
  - Amp of D50
    - 25g of Dextrose in a 50 ml 50% Solution of Dextrose
    - Used as IVP when glucose levels are very low, the patient is symptomatic and unable to safely eat.
  - Glucagon
    - If IV access is not available and or staff is having a difficult time obtaining IV access, Intramuscular Glucagon can be given to help bring glucose levels up. It acts on the liver to help release glucose stores.

- - Again, for hypoglycemia, only administered IM when there is no IV access for an Amp of D50 (I have only done this once or twice in my whole career so not very common)
  - A very common side of effect of glucagon is nausea and vomiting. Keep this in mind and be prepared to deal with the vomiting and any airway issues it may cause. (Turn them so they do not aspirate)
    - (Glucagon is also given for beta blocker OD. It will also cause nausea and vomiting. Give an antiemetic with it)
  - D5
    - Once the glucose level has been stabilized but continues to trend down. The patient may be started on a D5 drip/infusion to help maintain their glucose levels.
  - D10
    - If the D5 is not enough because the glucose is rapidly lowering, a D10 drip should be started to help maintain glucose levels.
- Nursing
  - Repeat Glucose check after interventions to ensure glucose is trending up.
  - If Glucose keeps trending down, let the team know so they can order additional D50 Amps and start them on an infusion of D5/D10/
  - Check a POC Glucose in your critical patients when they are decompensating and you can't figure out why.
  - When pushing an AMP of D50, if a small vein is used, push slowly, so you do not blow it as it will be a lot of pressure. Ideally a larger upper forearm and AC vein.

Diabetic Ketoacidosis

- A complication of diabetes mellitus where there is little to no insulin available to carry glucose into cells, leading to hyperglycemia. As the body is unable to use glucose for energy, it begins to break down fats, creating ketones as a by-product. Ketones are acidic and as they build up from fat breakdown, metabolic acidosis results. Hyperglycemia leads to osmotic diuresis, causing dehydration. The dehydration and metabolic acidosis lead to electrolyte abnormalities, and as the metabolic acidosis worsens organ dysfunction begins, ultimately, if left untreated, death.

- o The key issues are dehydration and electrolyte abnormalities from hyperglycemia and osmotic diuresis. As well as metabolic acidosis from ketones as a result of fat breakdown.
- o As a result patients will present with nausea, vomiting and abdominal pain as acid levels within the GI Tract are affected. Weakness and fatigue from impaired glucose use. Rapid breathing(kussmal) to help mediate acidosis by blowing off CO2. ALOC from a combination of the acidosis, dehydration, impaired glucose usage and electrolytes abnormalities. The classic symptoms are increased urination and increased thirst.
  - Ultimately, when severe, signs of shock such as hypotension and tachycardia will be present.
- o Causes include first onset diabetes mellitus, insulin noncompliance, infections, stress, trauma, alcohol binging and pancreas issues.
- Specifics of the workup
  - o Point of Care Glucose: To assess the level of glucose present. May read as 'high'
  - o Beta-Hydroxybutyrate (BHU): A ketone produced during fat breakdown. The higher the level, the worse off ketoacidosis is, prompting more aggressive management.
  - o CBC: Helps assess for infections. Infections can lead to a patient going into DKA.
  - o BMP: Helps assess electrolyte abnormalities and abnormalities with organs (Renal Function, Liver Labs, Pancreas and so forth)
    - Provides lab values necessary to calculate Anion Gap (Sodium - Chloride - Bicarb).
    - The anion gap is used to gauge the severity of acidosis. The body likes to stay in homeostasis, balancing cations(positive) and anions(negative), with a normal gap value being less than 12. When

there are outside substances like acidic ketones, the body becomes more acidic, raising the anion gap to levels greater than 12. As a result, we can calculate the anion gap to gauge how acidotic the body is.
- o Urinalysis: Help assess for ketones in the urine and possible sources of infection
- o Lactate: Assess for hypoperfusion as lactate is a byproduct of anaerobic metabolism, an indicator of poor perfusion to cells/organs
- o Infectious Workup if suspected: Chest Xray (pna etc), Blood Cultures, Urine Cultures, CT's (Remember the most common areas of severe infections are the chest, abdomen and pelvis)
- Treatment
  - o Fluid Administration: Normal Saline or Lactated Ringers
    - 30ml/kg or 1-2 L over 1 hour
    - Fluid administration helps treat the dehydration associated with osmotic diuresis and constant vomiting.
  - o Intravenous Insulin Therapy/Infusion: Key Treatment of DKA
    - *Only Regular Insulin can go IV*
    - Insulin will help cells use glucose for energy, stopping the breakdown of fats and production of ketones. This also reserves hyperglycemia, stopping osmotic diuresis.
    - Ensure potassium level is not low, if it is, it needs to be actively replaced while the insulin infusion is ongoing. Insulin drives potassium into cells, and if the levels are already low, it will cause further hypokalemia, which we know hypokalemia can be very irritating to the heart.
    - Check POC Glucose Hourly to monitor trend, ideally should be dropping 50-70 per hour. Also to ensure the patient does not go hypoglycemic while on the insulin infusion.

- Repeat BMP Q 4 hours to monitor electrolytes closely, as well as to calculate anion gap. (Sodium - Chloride - Bicarb)
  - Replace Electrolytes as needed
    - Potassium Level must be greater than 3.3 prior to starting insulin infusion
      - 10mEq peripherally per hour
      - 20mEq via central line per hour
      - PO: 40 mEq (PO pills are large, hard to swallow and can irritate the stomach, causing nausea)
    - Replace magnesium as it helps maintain potassium levels
  - Treat underlying cause if present
    - A big one here is infections. Locate source, culture if possible and administer antibiotics.
- Transitioning to SubQ Insulin / Resolved Ketoacidosis
  - Several criteria need to be met for the patient to be able to come off the insulin infusion
    - Anion gap less than 12
    - Bicarb >18
    - Pt is able to tolerate PO food intake
  - Once criteria are met, a long acting insulin is administered. The infusion remains ongoing for 2 hours after it was administered, then it can be discontinued. The long acting is administered concurrently to prevent hyperglycemia since it could easily throw the patient back into DKA.
- Nursing
  - Ask questions regarding possible precipitating sources like infections. Symptoms such as fever, chills, cough, sore throat, wounds and dysuria. Infections promote stress in the body, can cause electrolytes issues and the body naturally increases levels of glucose. For diabetics this is a perfect recipe for dka.
  - GAP calculation: Sodium - Chloride - Bicarb
  - Recheck glucose after fluid resuscitation (Prior to starting infusion infusion)
  - Insulin Infusion
    - Only Regular Insulin can go IV

- Wait for potassium level prior to start IV Insulin(Shifts potassium into cells, may need to replace it at the same time to prevent any cardiac effects)
- Check glucose hourly
- Repeat BMP q 4 hours to monitor electrolytes and calculate gap
  - Have at least 2 IV'S. One will be for the insulin infusion, while the others can be used for fluids and possible electrolyte replacements.
  - For nausea, reglan works better than zofran in diabetic patients as it promotes gastric emptying and gastric mobility, which are often problems dka patients have
  - IV Potassium is irritating to veins. Try to use a larger vein, or slow down rate or dilute with another normal saline infusion at a slow rate (per provider order)
    - Remember potassium IV is only 10 meQ per hour if peripheral, 20 mEq if central line.

Hyperkalemia

- Hyperkalemia is elevated potassium in the blood, with levels above 6mEq/L being concerning as high potassium can disrupt the electrical activity of the heart, leading to deadly arrhythmias.
  - Causes include kidney failure, missing dialysis, burns, rhabdomyolysis and certain medications such as potassium sparing diuretics. However, you'll most commonly deal with hyperkalemia with renal issues. Another cause can be cell breakdown from an inadequate blood draw (prolonged tourniquet use, slow flow, using a syringe).
  - Symptoms can include arrhythmias, ECG changes (Peaked T waves, Widening QRS), muscle weakness, fatigue, nausea and vomiting. Hyperkalemia is also commonly found on routine lab work, pt are told to go to the ER.
- Specifics of the workup: These patients often have other complaints that require additional and more in depth workups. For Hyperkalemia, the workup goes as follows:

- o Complete Metabolic Panel: Assess electrolytes including potassium. Assess kidney function as the kidneys are in charge of maintaining electrolyte balances, especially potassium.
- o ECG: Assess for any ECG changes indicative of hyperkalemia such as peaked T waves and a widening QRS. Also to assess whether any arrhythmias are present as that indicates the heart may already be irritated from the high levels of potassium
- o CBC: To ensure nothing is missed like an elevated white count or a low hemoglobin
- o Urinalysis: To assess renal function and any abnormalities
- Treatment
  - o Calcium Gluconate
    - Stabilizes the cardiac membrane, reducing heart irritability from potassium, helping prevent arrhythmias
    - 1 gram over 10 minutes
    - If hyperkalemia is causing instability and arrhythmias, I've seen up to 3 grams given initially.
  - o Insulin and Glucose
    - Insulin drives potassium into the cell, reducing extracellular potassium
    - Since insulin will also lower glucose levels, an amp of Dextrose is also given
    - 10 Units of Regular Insulin are typically given IV. If the glucose is already low prior to insulin administration, notify the providers and they may change to 5 Units, especially in renal patients, as the kidneys are incharge of clearing insulin.
  - o Sodium Bicarb
    - Shifts potassium into cells. Acidosis causes cells to release potassium while alkalosis causes cells to take in potassium. Bicarb is given to help create alkalosis, causing potassium to shift into cells
    - 50mEq (an amp) is typically given IV
  - o Kayexalate

- Binds potassium in the GI tract which is ultimately excreted. This helps maintain potassium levels within adequate levels
- Kayexate is important to give, however, it does take 4-6 hours to begin working so prioritize the above medications first.
  - Other medications can include
    - Albuterol
      - Shifts potassium inside cells. Consult with provider if the patient is tachycardic as albuterol will further increase the HR
    - Lasix
      - Helps increase potassium excretion by kidneys
      - Ensure the patient produces urine prior to administration, if they do not produce urine there is no point in administration. This is mainly for dialysis patients.
    - IV fluids
      - To dilute blood and as a result lower concentration of potassium
  - Dialysis
    - Key treatment for severe hyperkalemia. Dialysis will remove excess potassium.
    - Providers will need to place an emergency large bore catheter and dialysis department/RN would need to be readily available
- Nursing
  - Calcium Gluconate (Not Chloride-only for codes)
    - Give the calcium gluconate first so it begins to stabilize the heart. As it is infusing, you can work on gathering other medications.
  - Kayexalate is important, however, prioritize other meds first since it can take up to 6 hours to start working
  - Only Regular Insulin can go IV
  - Recheck poc glucose within 30 minutes to ensure glucose levels are maintaining since you most likely gave insulin

- A VBG can yield a potassium result rapidly compared to waiting for the bmp. Although you will still get a BMP, getting a VBG for the potassium can be useful
- Keep these patients on a cardiac monitor

Alcohol Withdrawal and Delirium Tremens

- Alcohol withdrawal occurs when a patient who regularly consumes large amounts of alcohol suddenly stops or reduces the amount of alcohol intake. Alcohol is a downer, it suppresses. To compensate for the suppression, the body becomes more excitable to counterbalance the suppressive effects of alcohol. When the alcohol intake suddenly stops, the body's compensatory mechanisms of increasing excitability are still present, and without alcohol to balance it out, the body becomes increasingly excitable.
    - As a result if every body system is ramped up, patients present with anxiety, irritability, combativeness, diaphoresis, nausea, tachycardia, hypertensive, hyperthermia, tremors, seizures and even hallucinations.
    - It can ultimately be deadly as a result of dehydration, electrolytes abnormalities, metabolic acidosis, arrhythmias, seizures and even as a result of being a danger to themselves.
- Specifics of the workup
    - Point of care glucose: common in alcohol withdrawal as these patients typically do not eat appropriately
    - Complete Metabolic Panel: Assess for electrolyte abnormalities. Assess renal function and liver function, which can be damaged from chronic alcohol use. The kidneys can be damaged from acute dehydration
    - CBC: Ensure issues like infections or low hgb are not missed.
    - Urine Toxicology: To assess for drug use which may be the cause of the current symptoms
    - Serum Alcohol Level
    - Coagulation study: As the liver plays an important role in clotting, it may be ordered to assess whether there are any issues or when suspected if hbg is low

- ECG: Assess for arrhythmias which can be predisposed from electrolyte issues or from the heart being overly excitable
- CT Head: Rule out other causes for confusion and hallucinations
- CIWA Assessment: Helps provide a numerical value for the severity of symptoms associated with withdrawal. The higher, the worst symptoms are and the more aggressive management should be.
  - Includes Nausea and vomiting, tremors, sweating, anxiety, agitation, hallucinations, headaches, and mentation/confusion.
- Treatment
  - Quiet environment and sitter
    - A sitter is often required to help prevent the patient from accidentally harming themselves as a result of their confusion and hallucinations
  - IV fluids
    - To help correct dehydration as a result of vomiting, diaphoresis and poor oral fluid intake by patient
  - Dextrose
    - Will be as an infusion with IV fluids as needed
  - Thiamine, Folic Acid and Vitamins
    - Help prevent wernicke's encephalopathy and help correct deficiencies present from chronic alcohol use
  - Electrolyte Replacement
    - Fix electrolyte abnormalities as indicated
  - Benzodiazepines
    - Common 1st line medications. They help alleviate withdrawal symptoms as they calm the body and nervous system, taking the place of alcohol. They work on GABA, an inhibitory neurotransmitter, just as alcohol does.
    - In mild to moderate cases, patients will get a scheduled dose of Lorazepam given, typically PO. Depending on the CIWA score, they may get an additional dose of Lorazepam to help alleviate symptoms. If the CIWA score continues to remain

high and or is trending up, and the patient is needing more IV Pushes of Lorazepam, the patient will be upgraded to ICU status and a Lorazepam drip may be ordered.

- If on a Lorazepam drip, close monitoring is essential to monitor for respiratory depression and improvement of symptoms. Place the patient on end tidal CO_2.

o Phenobarbital

- When patients are not responding to Lorazepam, phenobarbital should be added to help increase effects on GABA. Hence, further helping reduce the overexcitability present in the body.
- It will be administered IV, typically with an infusion of 10-15 minutes, depending on the dosing. I typically will place the phenobarb into a 50ml or 100ml NS bag, and infuse it over 10-15 minutes. Check with your facility for administration, however, typically you do not want to infuse faster than 60mg/min.

o Additional Medications that may be used

- Dexmedetomidine
  - Adjunct therapy used in combination with Lorazepam. It is typically used for its sedative effects, which is essential when patients are very aggressive, combative and confused.
  - Close monitoring is ideal as it can cause bradycardia. While using, I've had patients go really brady before, so please keep bradycardia at the back of your mind when starting Precedex (Dexmedetomidine).
- Propranolol
  - Used to help with autonomic hyperactivity (tachycardia and hypertension). Adjunct therapy, it should never replace appropriate dosing of Benzos and phenobarbital.

- Antipsychotics
    - Typically not used as they lower the seizure threshold and have effects on QT intervals, predisposing patients to arrhythmias. However, they may be ordered for severe agitation and confusion.
- Nursing
    - CIWA: Learn to calculate and what it entails
    - Check a POC Glucose
    - Multiple IV's and ideally in the forearm (so patient does not have to be reminded to straightened their arm). You will be giving fluids, replacing electrolytes, giving benzos and patients may pull them out due to confusion.
        - Cover IV's to help prevent patient removing
    - Communication with the managing provider/team is crucial as these patients when critical will need many doses of benzos and or additional medications. So promptly communicate when the CIWA is worsening or if the patient is becoming more confused and a danger to themselves and others or if vital signs are changing
    - Seizure padding should be placed
    - If on Lorazepam drip, place the patient on end tidal CO2 to help closely monitor respiratory status.

Atrial Fibrillation with a rapid ventricular response

- Mini patho: Atria contract irregularly and rapidly -> poor filling of ventricles -> fast electrical signals to ventricles -> ventricles contract rapidly, hence heart rate increases -> poor filling and rapid heart rate -> decreased cardiac output
- Nursing recognition: Recognition of afib on an ecg combined with a high heart rate, hypotension, palpitations, chest discomfort, sob
- Complications: Blood clots -> strokes, cardiomyopathy, hypotension -> syncope
- Essentials
    - Treat underlying condition (Sepsis, ACS, hyperthyroidism,

pulmonary embolisms etc)

- o Cardioversion (Onset within 48 hours, unstable, Transesophageal echocardiogram evaluating for blood clot within atria or is patient on blood thinners)
- o Fluids, Diltiazem or metoprolol, amiodarone, esmolol, magnesium, digoxin, cardiology consult
- o Monitor closely: repeat blood pressures often
- o Give medications slowly
- o Multiple IV's
- o Getting an ecg should be among the top of your to do list

Anaphylaxis

- Mini patho: Immune system overreacts to an allergen -> inflammatory mediators are released -> deadly effects seen in the respiratory and cardiovascular systems -> bronchoconstriction and low blood pressure -> respiratory and cardiovascular collapse
- Nursing recognition: Angioedema, Itchiness, Hives, Tachycardia, SOB, wheezing/stridor, dizziness
  - o Common causes: Food allergies, medications, contrast, stings, blood transfusions
  - o Questions: Ask about their allergies and possible triggers? Has this happened before? Has the patient needed to be intubated in the past? New Medications? Was epi already given and how long ago?
- Essentials
  - o Remove allergen
  - o ABC's
  - o Epinephrine IM (Epi pen should be readily available), IV, Fluids, Oxygen
  - o Other meds to help with symptoms: Diphenhydramine, H2 Blockers, Steroid, Albuterol
  - o Be prepared for a cricothyrotomy if pt needs to be intubated

Symptomatic Bradycardia

- Mini patho: HR < 50's (Sinus brady, Blocks etc) -> decreased cardiac output -> hypotension -> dizziness, altered, fatigued, sob, chest pain -> symptoms rise out of poor perfusion to body
- Essentials
  - IV, Oxygen, Monitor, Crash cart and pacing depending on rhythm, ECG
  - Medications: Atropine, Epinephrine, Calcium Gluconate, Glucagon/Zofran, High dose insulin/Dextrose
  - Figuring out cause: Too much beta blocker? Or Calcium Channel Blocker? 3rd degree AV block? Digoxin toxicity?

Aggressive / Violent Behavior

- **Your safety is a priority.** You won't be able to help the patient in front of you or any patient, if you become seriously hurt.
- The patient's safety is also an important priority. This may include not allowing them to further hurt themselves, assisting them in regaining control and ensuring we assess for and treat any medical issue found such as Intoxication, Seizure Postictal, Hepatic Encephalopathic, Head Injuries, Electrolyte issues and so forth. There can be countless causes for why the patient lost their sense of control.
- Patients who are irritated or upset but are still in their right mind will respond to good skills in de-escalation. The ER is busy, wait times can be long, they may be in pain, may be anxious, the average person will get irritated. Do not take it personal.
  - **Always maintain a safe distance** (Any patient is capable of violence)
  - **Remain calm and composed**. I know this can be difficult, we are human. The ED may be short staffed, you may not have even gotten a chance to use the restroom yet or even eat a snack. **But if we respond with frustration, it usually just escalates the situation**.
  - **Show Empathy and Listen Actively:** Demonstrate that you are genuinely listening by repeating back what the patient has said. My go to is, "I hear you." Building rapport is key, so you could also say something like, "That sounds very frustrating. Let's figure this out together. Here's what I can do right now."
  - **Focus on How You Can Help and Offer Simple Choices:** While you may not have control over certain things like wait times, you can provide assistance in other ways. For example, you could offer an ice pack, message the provider on their behalf, check where they are in the process, find them a place to sit, or even offer a meal. Direct towards that things you do have control over. **But if**

we respond with frustration, it usually just escalates the situation.

- o **Set Clear Boundaries and Don't Hesitate to Call Security:** Never allow the patient to block your exit. It's important to remember that any patient is capable of violence, so always stay aware of your surroundings. If a patient is yelling or using abusive language, calmly say, "I understand how upsetting this can be. I'm trying to help you, so please lower your voice so we can talk, and I can understand the situation." If they continue, while staying mindful of your environment, calmly but firmly ask them again to lower their voice. Let them know that if they are unable to do so, security will be called. Despite common culture as just part of the job, no one should ever be aggressive with you. Don't put up with it.

- Patients who are not in control of themselves may most likely not respond to de-escalation techniques. If they are aggressive, not receptive to de-escalation techniques and showing signs of escalation like pacing back and forth with fists clenched and actively stating that they are going to hurt you, you MUST call security for back up. Let the provider know after security. They may try different de-escalation techniques or just the fact that there is more personnel may persuade the patient to sit down and listen and perhaps choose and agree to medications.

  - o The situation may further escalate and turn into a take down where the patient is four point restrained and given antipsychotics/sedatives. **When restraining, to help avoid injury to staff and patient, you need a minimum of 6 people.** One person at each limp, one person to help ensure the patient is not biting or spitting and one person actively placing the restraints. It should be one arm up and one arm down and legs spread apart.

  - o It is important these patients also receive antipsychotics and sedative medications to help them relax because if they don't, they will continue to fight against the restraints and further injure themselves.

- **Medications** ordered to help calm/sedate these patients will vary from provider to provider, but they should keep in mind the cause of the agitation. Antipsychotics should be administered when schizophrenia, bipolar or delirium are suspected as the cause of the agitation, while benzodiazepines can be used when the agitation is as a result of alcohol withdrawal and intoxication with uppers (meth, PCP etc).

- o You'll find that in violent patients where rapid sedation is needed, both types of medications are ordered. You'll come across the phrase **B52**. Stands for **Benadryl 50mg, Haldol 5mg and Lorazepam 2mg**. (There are providers that may order Olanzapine 5-10mg instead of the haldol). In acute agitation, these medications **are going to be given Intramuscularly (IM)**. It is very difficult to place an IV on a patient that is combative and that is the perfect recipe for a needle stick injury.
- o **Benadryl**: Although an antihistamine, it does have sedative effects and it helps prevent EPS symptoms from administering Haldol (or Olanzapine)
- o **Haldol**: A first generation antipsychotic commonly used for agitation. A key potential side effect of haldol is that it can cause QT Prolongation and in susceptible patients that can lead to Torsades De Pointes.
- o **Lorazepam**: A benzodiazepine, a sedative. One of its many uses includes administration for acute agitation in combination with other medications like Haldol. A key side effect is respiratory depression.
- o **KEY NURSING POINT:** After giving medications, you must be very vigilant and closely monitor the patient. When these drugs are combined together, their potential for adverse effects intensify. These adverse effects include respiratory depression and ECG changes. As soon as you are able to safely do so, place the patient on the monitor spo2, ecg, BP, RR, Capno. If your combative verbal patient suddenly goes quiet, please be alarmed and go to assess and place on the monitor. This is very important when you've had to redose patients multiple times, all the medications can suddenly take effect together and cause respiratory depression.
  - ▪ **After the patient is sedated, do not lag in performing or obtaining the ordered tests. Do them while the patient is sedated. These**

include the ECG, going to CT, drawing labs, giving additional medications and so forth.

- With that in mind, if a patient is not cooperative and may become violent, do not attempt any intervention that may lead to personal injury such as lab draw. Discuss with the provider the potential for injury and if need be, state that you feel unsafe performing a task on a patient who may move and or cause injury to you. If the patient is borderline, discuss the use of PO medications while offering the patient food. When they take effect and the patient is more cooperative, then you can safely perform interventions.

- **Other Medications** include Olanzapine, Ziprazidone, Droperidol, Versed and Ketamine. Again, unless your facility has specific guidelines or protocols for acute agitation, the medications of choice for acute violent behavior will be provider choice. **Your job is to ensure your safety and the patients safety.**
  - o **Olanzapine**: A second generation antipsychotic that can be used for acute agitation. Common first dose is 5-10 mg IM. Side effects include hypotension, QT prolongation and oversedation (closely monitor when combining with other medications).
  - o **Ziprasidone**: A second generation antipsychotic that can be used for acute agitation. Common first dose is 10-20mg. The Key Issue with Ziprasidone is its potential for QT Prolongation and ultimate torsades de pointes. As with haldol, careful use of it in patients with ecg/cardiac issues.
  - o **Droperidol**: An antipsychotic that can be used for acute agitation. Common dose is 5-10mg IM. Key side effect is QT prolongation and as a result deadly rhythms.
  - o **Midazolam**: A benzodiazepine with strong sedative properties that can be used for acute violent behavior. Dosing is 2.5-5mg IM. Key side effects include respiratory depression, oversedation and hypotension.
  - o **Ketamine**: A dissociative anesthetic with potent sedative properties. I've typically seen ketamine ordered for the very severe violent patients who've typically come back positive with multiple substances on the tox screen like PCP and

meth. The dosing Intramuscularly may seem like a lot, it is 4-5mg/kg **IM(Intramuscular).** Key side effects include emergence reactions (confusion when waking up), increase in HR and BP, and in rare occasions laryngospasm(may have to intubate).

- o **Nursing Key Point:** Closely monitor your patients after administering any of these medications. Watch out for oversedation, respiratory depression, hypotension and QT prolongation. Place on the cardiac monitor with continuous SPO2, BP, RR, HR, ECG and even end tidal CO_2. In emergency situations with acute agitation, these medications **are going to be given IM.**

- **Charting Tips:** Ensure your charting supports the use of restraints and sedative medications. Clearly state why these interventions were performed including the patients behavior, abusive language, physical attacks that were made by the patient and so forth.
  - o Include the least restrictive methods that were used first including therapeutic communication, de-escalation techniques, offering PO medications, offering food and so forth. Include how the patient was at risk of hurting others and hurting themselves.
  - o When charting about restraints ensure to include the type, where they were placed, assessments of the placement sites, and constant evaluation for the need of restraints. Plus how you assessed for injury, pain, need for restroom use, water, food etc.
  - o Chart when and how the provider was made aware and the orders given

  - o Ensure your documentation is in line with the policies of your facility

Medications

With medications, #1 is

- **Always ask about allergies before giving any medication.** Once it's in the body, you can not take it back. Always ask for allergies.

Although all medications deserve your undivided attention, you need to be extra careful with **insulins, opioids, blood thinners, blood pressure meds, and any medication that you are giving to a pediatric patient.**

- **Blood Thinners**
  - What is the reason for the medication? Is it for atrial fibrillation, a PE or DVT, for a stent, or for DVT prophylaxis?
  - Do you need to have baseline coags? Ideally, yes. Even for DVT prophylaxis. It helps assess for any undiagnosed coagulation disorders.
  - Are they going to surgery any time soon? If they are, always consult with the provider to ensure it is safe to continue. They would have to take into consideration the risks of thrombotic events and potential bleeding.
  - Are they currently bleeding from anywhere? Ask about blood in their stool (black or red), blood in vomitus (red or coffee ground) and assess for significant bruising throughout their body. If this patient is going to be admitted to the hospital, they should have had a CBC, what is the HGB/HCT.
- **Insulins**
  - What is the Point of Care Glucose? It needs to be recent, no more than 30-45 minutes old.
  - Is the patient insulin naive? If so, ensure the provider is aware and recheck a Point of Care Glucose based on the onset and peaks. Also monitor for signs of hypoglycemia such as diaphoresis, confusion, tachycardia and so forth.
  - Do you know how to treat hypoglycemia? Review hypoglycemia in section on Common Conditions
- **Blood Pressure Lowering Medications**
  - Always check the blood pressure before administering. If it is on the lower side, notify your provider before

administration to ensure they still want it. If it is less than 90, never administer. Notify your provider.
- o Be mindful of orthostatics. If your patient has to get up, do it slowly. Have them sit at the edge of the bed for a few minutes first, then stand slowly with you always present.
- **IV Opioids**
    - o Always give very slowly. Never Fast IV Push. If needed dilute with normal saline in order to give it more slowly and in a controlled manner.
    - o Double verify dosing. Be mindful of the dosing in elderly and pediatrics.
    - o Are they on a monitor? Have they ever had IV opioids before? Is oxygen equipment readily available if needed? For peds, always double check the dosing with a buddy nurse.

Again, always ask for help if you do not know something or if you feel unsure about anything, especially when it comes to medications.

<u>Vasopressors</u>: See section on vasopressors.

<u>ACLS Medications</u>: See Section on ACLS Meds

<u>BP Lowering Meds:</u> See treatment of Hypertensive Emergency

<u>Rapid Sequence Intubation Medications</u>

Sedative before Paralytic! Always. The main sedative used is Etomidate, while the two main paralytics are Roccuroneum and Succinylcholine.

- **Etomidate**
    - o Primary Sedative used as it is hemodynamically stable and has a fast onset. It will not lower blood pressure or increase the heart rate.
    - o Onset: 10-30 seconds. Duration: 5-10 minutes.
    - o Dosing: Commonly 0.3mg/kg
    - o Side Effects
        - ▪ Besides respiratory depression(which is fine since the patient is getting intubated), it can cause myoclonus (seizure like jerking movements),

although it is typically self limiting and will go away on its own. Just nice to know about it.

- **Succinylcholine**
  - o Paralytic commonly used as it works fast and does not last long. In Rapid Sequence Intubation when a patient needs to be intubated in a safe yet rapid manner, a paralytic that works fast is ideal. If the intubation is unsuccessful and or there are complications, it is beneficial that it wears off fast so the patient can regain the ability to breath on their own which reduces potential prolonged hypoxia and gives the team time to come up with alternative techniques such as video laryngoscope or even calling the anesthesia team for assistance if available.
  - o Onset: 30-60 seconds. Duration: up to 10 minutes
  - o Dosing is typically 1.5mg/kg
  - o Side Effects
    - ▪ The key disadvantage of succs is that it can cause **hyperkalemia** so it is avoided in renal patients, burns, crush injuries, rhabdomyolysis and any condition where hyperkalemia would be a concern.
    - ▪ It can also cause malignant hypertension
- **Rocuronium**
  - o Paralytic used when Succs is not ideal. Although it typically does not have contraindications like succs, it is not primary used due to its longer onset and duration.
  - o Onset: up to 2 minutes. Duration: up to 60 minutes
  - o Dosing is typically 1mg/kg
  - o Side Effects
    - ▪ Although no major contraindication, be prepared to handle unsuccessful intubations due to its prolonged duration of 1 hour. Have BVM with NPA/OPA readily available or even a supraglottic airway. (Even supplies needed for emergency cric).
    - ▪ If needed, the reversal agent is Sugammadex.
- **Ketamine**
  - o Although not commonly used as a sedative for intubation, it still has important uses. Key points of ketamine include that patients typically maintain their respiratory drive, it has bronchodilatory effects, can increase heart rate and blood

pressure, and it has analgesic properties. Therefore, it can be a good option for when asthmatics or COPD patients need to be intubated. Also useful for high risk Awake Intubations.

- Onset: 30-60 seconds. Duration: 10-20 minutes
- Dosing for RSI is typically 1.5mg/kg
- Side Effects

  - It is not used as often as it comes with the risk of laryngospasm, increased cerebral edema and as a result of increasing the heart rate, it can place further strain on a weakened heart.

Heart Rate Medications

- Intravenous **Diltiazem**(Cardizem):
  - A calcium channel blocker used to lower heart rate. Used primarily IV in the ER with Atrial Fibrillation with a rapid ventricular response. At times, providers may also use it for SVT.
  - Dosing: 0.25mg/kg. Typically for adults most providers will just order around 20mg IV
    - Usually followed by 30mg PO tablet to help control the heart rate longer.
  - Admin and Side Effects: Don't Push it. Give it slowly over two minutes. Cycle the bp right before it, during and after to ensure it did not drop a significant amount.
    - If the BP is already low beforehand, do not give it until you talk to the provider about it. Perhaps start a liter of NS prior to administration of Diltiazem. If the BP is low, and you give it, it will only make it go lower. (They may tell you that the BP will go up after the heart rate comes down due to better filling of the ventricles and so forth but if the BP is already low beforehand, don't administer until the BP is addressed first).
- **Intravenous Metoprolol**
  - A beta blocker used to lower heart rate. Typically used intravenously for atrial fibrillation with a rapid ventricular response.

- o Dosing: 2.5-5 mg slow IV. Can be repeated. If it works, typicallyed followed by a PO dose of 50mg for longer hear rate control.
- o Side Effects
    - Like with cardizem, do not administer if the BP is low, address the BP first.
    - Should not be used with patients who have asthma or COPD due to possibility of bronchoconstriction
- **Intravenous Esmolol**
    - o A beta blocker to lower heart rate. Typically used as an infusion/drip. I have only used it for bringing the BP down in aortic dissections and for bringing the HR down in Afib RVR.
        - It slows the HR down, therefore decreasing cardiac output and BP.
        - Useful in Dissection because you don't just want to give a med that will only lower the BP, the body will response to this by increasing the HR and contractility, which will make the dissection worse. Esmolol helps with both bringing the HR down and BP.
    - o Fast on fast off. Onset within 1 minute and duration of only up to 9-10 minutes.
    - o The infusion will typically require a loading dose followed by 50mcg/kg/min, titrating by 50mcg/kg/min q 5-10mins, max of 200mcg/kg/min
    - o **(Please verify drips/infusions start rates, titrations, and max with your own facilities protocols)**
- **Intravenous Amiodarone**
    - o An antiarrhythmic that prolongs the actual potential which can help restore normal sinus rhythm or rate control by reducing the heart rate. Used for arrhythmias such as Ventricular tachycardia, Ventricular fibrillation and atrial fibrillation
    - o During cardiac arrest as with ventricular fibrillation or pulseless ventricular tachycardia
        - Dosing: 300mg IV push, if needed followed by a second dose of 150mg
    - o With atrial fibrillation or with a stable ventricular tachycardia
        - Loading Dose of 150mg IV over 10 minutes

- Followed by an infusion of 1mg/min over 6 hours (typically 360 mg)
- Then 0.5mg/kg infusion over 18 hours (typically 540 total)
  - Considerations
    - It can cause hypotension, bradycardia and QT prolongation.
    - If bradycardia is an issue, communicate with the team as it should not be used.
    - If your patient is hypotensive or on the lower side, discuss with the team. Set your BPs to repeat q5 minutes after starting drip/infusion for 30 minutes to assess how your patient responds.
    - Although typically not a concern in the ER, long term use can cause pulmonary, liver and thyroid toxicity.

Sedation and Analgesia for Intubated patients

- **Propofol**
  - A sedative hypnotic used for sedation of intubated mechanically ventilated patients.
  - A key feature of propofol is that it has a fast onset and short duration. "Fast on, Fast off." This makes it great for most patients especially neuro pts as an accurate neuro assessment can be obtained relatively quick after stopping the infusion.
    - Onset within 1 minute, duration up to 10 minutes. Except if it has been administered long term, allow up to 30 minutes for effects to fully wear off.
  - Range of 5-50mcg/kg/min (have seen higher ranges), with typical start of 5mcg/kg/min, titrated by 5mcg Q10 minutes. Some patients may need to be titrated or started with higher doses to maintain appropriate sedation, if so, ensure your provider is aware and provides an order to do so (since you may be going outside the set protocol). **Please review your facilities start dose, titration dose and interval and max range.**
  - Considerations

- It will cause respiratory depression and hypotension. Your pt is intubated so respiratory depression is not an issue typically. For hypotension, cycle BPs Q5 mins initially after starting infusion to ensure you closely monitor how your patient responds. If propofol drops the BP and is not maintaining adequate sedation, another agent should be used such as versed. (Sometimes providers want to use propofol for sedation for its fast off properties and may add a vasopressor such as Levophed to maintain the BP).
- Change the tubing every 12 hours to prevent bacterial growth.
- Do not let the bottle run empty! Ever! Your patient will wake up and try to take the ET Tube out.
- Propofol Infusion Syndrome: Extremely rare. Associated with high doses and prolonged use. Key characteristics are cardiovascular collapse and arrhythmias

- **Versed(Midazolam)**
  - Used as an infusion for sedation of intubated patients when pts are hemodynamically unstable (low bp:since prop can drop the bp significantly).
  - Onset is within 5 minutes and duration can be up to an hour. If the infusion has been long term, the duration may be significantly longer.
  - **For dosing, please review your organization's protocol.**
  - Considerations
    - Main issue is respiratory depression, if pt is intubated, typically not an issue.
    - At higher prolonged doses, it can cause hypotension. However, typically not as severe as propofol.
    - Reversal Agent: Flumazenil/Romazicon
- **Fentanyl**
  - Used as an infusion for pain management (opioid analgesic) for intubated patients. It is used in combination with Versed and or Propofol as either of those do not have any effects on pain.

- o **For dosing, please review your organization's protocol.**
- o Considerations
    - As with any opioid it can cause respiratory depression. With intubated patients, it is not an issue.
    - (When giving it for pain in non-intubated patients please dilute and give slow. If given fast, it will cause respiratory depression, hypotension and chest wall rigidity.)
- **Precedex**
    - o An alpha 2 agonists with mild sedative properties. Used when a mild/slight sedation is desired. The patient keeps their own respiratory drive and usually wakes up with physical stimulation.
    - o Onset is within 10 minutes. With duration, patients wake up almost immediately after discontinuing, but may feel drowsy for 1-2 hours.
    - o Considerations
        - It can cause bradycardia and hypotension, especially when a loading dose is given prior to starting the infusion.
            - This has happened quite a bit in the past when I have used precedex. If it does, stop the infusion, call the team and be prepared to administer IV fluids or atropine or a vasopressor as needed. (Typically after stopping it and giving a bolus of NS, the effects go away even by the team the team arrives)

Psych Acute Agitation Meds

- See section on Psych/Violent Patients: Ketamine, Ativan, Versed, Olanzapine, Risperidone, Benadryl, Haldol

Antidotes

- Acetaminophen- Acetylcysteine
- Digoxin-Digoxin Immune Fab

- Benzodiazepine-Flumazenil
- Heparin-Protamine Sulfate
- Organophosphates-Atropine and Pralidoxime
- Anticholinergics-Physostigmine
- Warfarin- Vitamin K / FFP / Prothrombin Complex Concentrate
- Ethylene Glycol and Methanol - Fomepizole
- Insulin - Glucose

Other important meds (Many of these are discussed in the common conditions section)

- Thrombolytics, Heparin, Calcium Gluconate, Glucagon, Regular Insulin, Phenobarbital, NS vs LR, Hypertonic Saline, Mannitol, Morphine, Fentanyl, Dilaudid, Octreotide, Dilantin, Valproic Acid, Furosemide, Metoclopramide, Meclizine, Aspirin, Ondansetron, GI cocktail, Protonix, Kayexalate

Laboratory Studies you MUST KNOW

Please review your own organization's lab value ranges

- *Lactate*: Commonly used in the ER to help assess a patient's perfusion status. It's a byproduct of anaerobic metabolism, meaning the body isn't getting the blood flow or oxygen it needs, so it turns to anaerobic metabolism and lactate is a result of it. The higher the lactate the worse the patients perfusion status may be. A normal lactate is less than 2 mmol/L. The higher the worst off the patient may be, and typically from what I've seen, lactate levels above 5 indicate a very sick patient.

- **D-Dimer**: When the body is breaking down a blood clot somewhere, D-Dimer is produced. The higher the D-Dimer that higher chances a blood clot is actually present, and many providers will use a cut off of 500ng/ml when it comes to pulmonary embolisms. If the patient has a D-Dimer above 500, then a ct scan with contrast will most likely be ordered to rule out or in a PE.

- **Ammonia**: A waste that is usually cleared by the liver and when there is a build up, it can result in patients presenting with altered mental status. Keep this in mind in patiens who have a history of liver failure and or chronic alcohol use. Normal is < 80 mcg/dL.

- **CBC**

  - **WBC**: white blood cells fight infections, if you have a high amount, there is an infection somewhere in the body. Normal is 4.5-10. Neutrophils are mature wbc's while bands are the immature version. When a patient has a bad infection and they start having a higher number of bands, its called a Left shift, indicating that the body is unable to keep up with the infection and is even throwing immature wbc's at it.

  - **Hemoglobin**: in the ER, commonly used to evaluate if a patient will need a blood transfusion. The typical threshold is that a hgb less than 7 g/dL will get a blood transfusion. Of course, this is a rule of thumb. If your patient is actively bleeding, their hemoglobin may not be low when the labs result because the body hasnt had to time to adjust and redistribute accordingly.

- ○ **Platelets**: clotting. If very low, less than 50, spontaneous bleeding can occur.

- **Coags**

  - ○ **Pt, INR, Ptt**: the body's overall clotting ability. Useful when patients are on blood thinners. Checked when patients are having any sort of bleed like a gi and intracranial bleed to ensure they don't need to be reversed.

- **Thromboelastography** (Teg)

  - ○ Body clotting ability but shown with specific clotting factors. Used in patients with severe bleeding to help decide if the patient needs more PRBC's, plasma, platelets or even cryo. It helps guide therapy.

- **BMP**

  - ○ **Electrolytes**
    - ■ **Sodium**
      - Hypernatremia: commonly as a result of Dehydration
      - Hyponatremia: commonly as a result of Volume Overload
      - Below 120s is critical r/t potential for seizures and other symptoms: key issue is to replace sodium slowly because if its done too fast a condition called osmotic demyelination syndrome can occur which essentially results in severe neuro symptoms.
    - ■ **Potassium**

- Hyperkalemia: commonly as a result of muscle breakdown and kidney injury/failure. Very toxic and irritating to heart muscle, so a level above 6 specially when combined with ecg changes needs to be treated asap.
- Hypokalemia: Commonly as a result of gastrointestinal and absorption disorders. Also irritating to the heart and needed by muscles to function, so levels below 3.5, but specially below 3, need to be replaced.

- **Calcium**
  - Important for cardiac conduction, so keep in mind when patients present with bradyarrhythmias
  - Will need to replace when patients receive multiple units of PRBC's
  - Keep in mind when patient is having arrhythmias

- **Magnesium**
  - Important for cardiac conduction and conduction throughout body
  - Keep in mind when patient is having arrhythmias

- **CO2**
  - Used interchangeably with the bicarb
  - Useful in determining if metabolic acidosis is present
  - Anion gap: Sodium - Chloride + CO2(BICARB)
    - Normal is between 10-12

- **Kidney**
  - Creatinine: used to assess kidney function. Greater than 1.5 kidney function is beginning to show compromise

- GFR: Helps assess kidney function, normal is greater than 90
- BUN: helps assess kidney function, 10-21 is normal
- **Liver**
  - ALT/AST: used to assess for liver dysfunction, the higher the worst off the liver is. ALT is more Liver specific
- **Pancreas**
  - Lipase/Amylase: used to assess function of pancreas, lipase is more specific.
- **Heart**
  - Troponin: useful in determining if heart damage is occurring, useful in patients potentially having a myocardial infarction
  - BNP: used to assess for heart failure. Normal bnp is 100 ng/L. A bnp >500 is typically a sign of a heart failure exacerbation. In my patient population, I commonly see Bnp's in the thousands.

- **Urine**
  - **Urine Tox Screen:** looks for illicit drugs like amphetamines and opioids
  - **Urinalysis**: measures and looks for a variety of things inside the urine like wbcs, nitrate, ketones, bacteria, blood, myoglobin, specific gravity, etc
  - **Urine Culture:** looks for bacteria in the urine

Blood Cultures: looks for bacteria in the blood and helps us figure out which abx would work best for the patient

Key Questions for Emergency Services

- Where did the patient come from? Who is the caregiver that knows about the patient? What is their name and phone number?

    o Sticky situations often come out of not knowing who to contact for more information about the patient. Especially for patients who are altered. Or what if the patient is getting discharged but you have no idea where they go back to or who to contact. So when your patients are older and or altered in any way, please ask for contact information.

- Is the patient full code? Is there a POLST?

    o Especially important for patients who are older and or those very critical . You want to ensure you honor their wishes if something comes up. The last thing you want is to start CPR or assist with intubating a patient who codes when they were actually a DNR/DNI.

- What is the patient's baseline? Mentation Baseline?

    o Although you can get information from the caregivers, in time sensitive situations like Strokes, ensuring you ask about the patient's baseline from emergency services is extremely important. You want to know what is new from what is old as it can help guide care and or with monitoring for improvement or worsening of patient condition.

- What medications did you give?

    o If the patient is coming in for chest pain, and it may be an ACS work up type of patient, did they give aspirin or nitroglycerin? Did the nitroglycerin help with the pain? For example, if they didn't give aspirin, you know you will most likely end up giving some. Or let's say the patient was having seizures and received benzo's enroute, you want to know how much and at what time. If the patient continues to be altered past the point of when the meds should have worn off, then it signals other issues may be going on.

- What is the blood sugar?
  - o Checking a point of care blood sugar on altered or comatose patients is one of the ER's most fundamental things to do to rule out hypoglycemia. So we want to ask just to ensure a check was already done, even though we will do our own. I remember I had a patient who came in crashing, and blood sugar was not checked enroute, and it ended up being low in the 20's.

- What is the chief complaint?
  - o Of course, although emergency services are really good at communicating their report, just ensure that at the end of the day you need a clear understanding of what the patient came in for.

History Taking: Questions and Information Gathering

Chief Complaint: What brings you in today? How can we help? Give the patient enough time to state their complaint in their own words. Then as you are getting a clear picture of the situation, direct the conversation to obtain the details you need.

Details of complaint: When did it start? Was it sudden or gradual? What were you doing when it started? What makes it worse or better? How do you describe the discomfort/pain? Where is it at and does it radiate? Have you had it before and what happened? What have you tried and did it help? If pain, how bad is it out of 10? Ask about associated symptoms for example if chest pain ask about dizziness, sob, nausea, or palpitations. If a headache ask about blurry vision or double vision, light sensitivity, dizziness, numbness or tingling sensations. If abdominal pain ask about nausea and vomiting, changes in stool, changes in urine.

History: Medical problems? What medications do they take? Changes in meds? Prior surgeries? Drugs? Alcohol? Smoker? Allergies?

ER Nursing in 1 2 3 : 3 Steps

To better help you process what is going on with your patients try to implement this 3 step process that I use.

- First, ask yourself what your patients issues/complaints/diagnosis are.
- Then, go over what you can anticipate for these issues. How can you be proactive?
- Finally, ask yourself, what the worst possible complications are? And how can you monitor for them or help prevent them?

Now, let's go over a few examples and how we can use the 3 step process.

Example 1: Your patient came in as a fentanyl overdose. He was found down, and needed several doses of narcan. Patient is now gcs 15, fully awake and alert, maintaining their airway and taking good deep breaths on their own. Last narcan dose given was 15 minutes ago just prior to the patient getting to you.

What are your patients issues? Overdosed on an opioid so his respiratory drive may be affected and can be at risk of respiratory failure if he stops breathing again. How can we be proactive? We can have narcan readily available just in case it's needed. We can also be proactive by placing the patient on endtidal co2 to help us more closely monitor that patient. We can also place the patient near the nurses station, where we have a direct line of sight to the patient. Complications? The main one is if the patient stops breathing. So how are we monitoring the patient and preventing it? Keeping a close eye on the patient and by placing endtidal co2 to help further assist with monitoring.

Example 2: Your patient has missed dialysis for a week, and is complaining of feeling increasingly tired.

What are their issues? Dialysis takes on the role of the kidneys, removing waste and extra fluids from the blood as well as a few other things. So they can have electrolyte issues or fluid overload, such as too much potassium or even fluid in the lungs that causes respiratory distress.

So how can we be proactive? We know that a high potassium can cause deadly arrhythmias, so we can start preparing to obtain an ECG. If the ECG is beginning to show ecg changes, it can guide treatment. We can also recommend sending a VBG, since it usually results fast and can have a rough potassium level. We know that the ultimate intervention is dialysis, so we can even give the dialysis RN a heads up. If the patient is in respiratory distress, it may be as a result of fluid buildup in the lungs, so we might anticipate noninvasive ventilation like bipap or cpap, so we can call RT and bring over the machine for them to set up.

So remember, what are the issues? How can we be proactive or what can we anticipate? And how do we monitor and prevent complications?

Focused Assessments

Why should we be good with our assessments? Well, in the ER, we are trying to rule out or look for diseases that are deadly! Differentiating patients who are sick vs not sick. As an ER nurse, you are going to be busy, you're going to have many things to do, and you need to figure out who deserves your time the most, aka prioritization.

So the goal is to be quick and concise! You should eventually get to the point where you are in and out in 5-10 mins or less! But of course, in this time you will find out if your patient is "sick" and if they are you will devote more time to them.

One point I want to make is that although we are only talking about the assessment here, it is important to know that you will be performing interventions and treatments while performing the assessment.

Respiratory Assessment

So what are we trying to answer when we are doing a respiratory assessment? We are focusing on the lungs, trying to figure out if adequate gas exchange is occurring, and gas exchange is determined by a fine balance between ventilation (air movement-oxygen) and oxygenation (blood absorbing oxygen).

Initial Assessment

The first part of the assessment is the visual assessment, otherwise known as the first or initial impression. I've heard it called the 'visual vital signs.' Here we are simply looking at the patient and determining if they look sick. Key findings include:

- Increased or decreased respiratory rate
- Use of accessory muscles
- Tripoding
- Audible stridor and wheezing
- Visible swelling of the lips or tongue

- Inability to speak.

Again, you can tell all of this from the door of the room, which is why it's known as the visual assessment.

Patient Who is Not III Appearing

If the patient isn't in severe respiratory distress and is able to speak, we'll gather information from them.

Questions

- When did the sob or difficulty breathing start?
- What were they doing? For example, just sitting down vs strenuous activity?
- Was it sudden? (Think of PE's or a spontaneous pneumo) (Side note, I've seen a lot of spontaneous pneumos in tall and skinny patients)
- Was the sob gradual?(perhaps pneumonia or chf exacerbation?)
- Do they experience sob or sensation of drowning with laying down or activity? (Cardiac issue like chf or anemia even).
- Ask if they have a cough, whether it is productive or not and if so, what color? Ask about fevers and chills? (Infectious sources of symptoms like pneumonia).
- Any recent airplane travel or long car rides where the patient is sitting? (DVT's -> PE's).
- Has this every happened before? What was done for it in the past?

Medical Hx and Medications

- Is there a history of lung issues such as COPD or Asthma?
- History of cardiac issues?
- What current medications are you taking? Keeping note of albuterol and other inhalants and meds like lasix, **are they even taking them?** They ran out? Can't afford them?
- Do they smoke or used to smoke? Smokers get lung damage so more at risk for pulmonary complications.

Physical Assessment:

- Respiratory Rate and Effort
- Chest Symmetry and Breathing Pattern
- Listen to lung fields: Comparing sides as you go. Assess for air movement (at least they are getting air/oxygen in and CO_2 out)
- Abnormal Lung Sounds: crackles(chf, pna) or wheezing(perhaps asthma or allergic reaction), or rhonchi (pna, copd).
- Listen to trachea if needed for stridor: may indicate a partial upper airway obstruction
- SPO2

Patient Who is Ill Appearing

Your initial impression tells you that this patient is sick.
Your patient may not be able to speak and answer questions. When this occurs, treatments take priority (while simultaneously assessing).

Immediate Actions

- Place on cardiac monitor: SPO2, Respiratory Rate, ECG, Heart Rate, BP
- Provide oxygen: Depending on the severity use Nasal Cannula, Non-rebreather (NRB) or bag-valve mask (BVM)
- Obtain IV access: Crucial for medications

You're part of a team, so it may be your provider assessing while you're focused on the tasks above.
If you are working alone,

1) First, place on oxygen and ensure someone is notifying the provider.
2) Second, Place the patient on the pulse ox, then listen to their lungs, assessing for air movement.
   a) If the patient is working really hard to breathe but there isn't air movement, the patient can go into respiratory failure shortly.

Continue Stabilization/Assessment

- Listen to the lungs: crackles, wheezing, stridor
- Connect your patient onto the rest of the cardiac monitor to obtain vital signs and basic ECG rhythm

- As far as vital signs, if the patient is tachy and has one swollen lower ext then possible PE? Tachy and fever, then pneumonia ? If spo2 is not improving on a NRB or with BVM, then does the patient need to go on noninvasive(bipap/cpap) or get intubated? *Keeping in mind that for bipap/cpap mentation needs to be intact so pt can protect their own airway.*

- Assess for Respiratory Effort, Retractions, chest wall symmetry (equal chest rise and fall), patient position (ex tripoding), skin color and pt alertness/mentation.
  - If mentation is declining and there is minimal air movement on auscultation, respiratory failure is imminent.

- Assess for edema to lower extremities, abdomen and upper extremities, is it possibly chf or liver failure? Any vomit around face or clothing, signaling perhaps aspiration? Edema or swelling of lips and tongue will lead you to an anaphylactic reaction.

- Do they need respiratory medications? Albuterol and Atrovent breathing treatment to open airways? Magnesium to help relax bronchial smooth muscle? Steroids to decrease inflammation in the airways? Prioritize these medications.

Then after assessment and interventions are underway you can start on history gathering, whether from EMS, family, patient, or a chart review.

Cardiac Assessment

With the cardiac assessment, we are trying to figure out if the body is getting the perfusion it needs.

Initial Impression

With the Initial Impression, we are looking for:

- Mottled skin, diaphoresis, paleness, level of consciousness, patient position, and whether they are guarding or clenching at their chest.

Questions

- Assess Orientation
  - What is your name?
  - What year is it? What month is it?
  - Where are you right now?
  - What brought you to the ER?
  - These essentially tell you that the patient is having adequate perfusion to the brain at this moment in time and is able to think and recall.
- Question Chest Pain Symptoms
  - Does your chest hurt? Or do you feel pressure or palpitations?
    - I've found that some patients don't consider pressure pain, and if you just ask about pain they may not bring up palpitations either. You can ask if their heart is racing instead of using the work palpitation.
  - When did your chest pain start?
  - What were you doing? Were you up and around doing activities or were you resting or were you eating?
  - Where is your pain? Does it radiate? Does it go to your shoulders, arms, back, neck or jaw?
  - What makes it worse? Does activity make it worse? What makes it better? Does rest make it better?
  - Is the pain constant or does it come and go?
  - Another important question is whether this type of pain has happened before, how did it go away and if they went to seek medical help, what were they told?
- Associated Symptoms
  - Dizziness, sob, nausea/vomiting and weakness which can all point to a cardiac etiology.

Medical History and Medications
- Any diagnosed heart problems? Any prior heart attacks?
- What medications are they currently on?

- o Are they on blood thinners? Bp meds? Aspirin on a daily basis?
- Risk Factors: Smoking, Obesity, HTN, prior MI's. Essentially the more risks factors the likelihood something serious is occurring increases.
- **Key Point:** Diabetic patients and women may present with nonspecific discomforts when having myocardial ischemia, so consider at least an ECG in these patients.
- **Key Point:** This brings me to a very a important point, which is that an ECG needs to be completed within 15 mins of pt arrival, or it at least should be among the top things of your to do list because it can show an MI, arrhythmias, and even give clues for a PE.
- Now, what about drug use? Drugs like cocaine and meth can cause cp from how hard they make the heart work. It's important to ask because treatment may differ.

Physical Assessment

- Cardiac Monitor
  - o Blood Pressure, Hear Rate, Spo2, Cardiac Rhythm
  - o I always like to repeat my patients blood pressure right off the bat even if the first one is great, especially if they "look" sick, I just don't fully trust the monitors.
  - o Having the rhythm on the monitor is helpful because you can quickly see if your patient is in SVT, or afib rvr, or even in V-tach.
  - o Tachycardia with a low blood pressure is indicative of shock. The heart rate rises to compensate.
- Skin color, Pulses and Capillary Refill
  - o A useful rule of thumb is that an SBP of around 70 is needed for carotid and femoral pulses to be palpable, while approximately an sbp of 80 is needed for a radial pulse and an sbp of 100 for pedal pulses. So if you can feel a radial pulse, you know that the bp is at least in the 80's or above. This is useful if the patient is not yet on the monitor or when

the monitor is unable to capture a blood pressure.

   o A cap refill greater than two is considered delayed.
- Edema: Is it bilateral or unilateral? Bilateral tends to be a heart issue while unilateral can be a venous issue, perhaps a DVT. Take a quick look assessing for JVD as it can be a quick way of assessing for fluid overload, besides obvious pitting edema in the lower extremities.
- Auscultate: Keep it simple. Are heart sounds loud and clear? Or are they distant? Irregular? Do you hear extra heart sounds like S3 S4 or murmurs?

Further assessments that can occur at the bedside include a bedside echocardiogram performed by your provider.

As far as history, if the patient cannot provide it, you'll do your best to obtain it from family, friends, EMS, and or a chart review if the patient has been at your facility in the past.

Keeping it simple, the cardiac assessment will include:
- Level of consciousness
- ECG
- Vitals: BP, HR, RR, SPO2
- Skin color, pulses, cap refill
- Symptoms: Chest pain, Chest Pressure, Palpitations, SOB, nausea/vomiting, diaphoresis, dizziness, Pale

Neuro Assessment

Time is brain! You do not want to be the nurse who missed a code stroke while triaging. You also want to accurately trend your patients assessment throughout the shift, to ensure you catch changes.

As we know, the first sign of deterioration in a neuro patient will be their mentation and level of consciousness. This will happen way before you start noticing vital sign changes and or pupil changes. By obtaining a thorough baseline assessment, you can compare down the line when something changes. For example, if your patient is requiring more stimulation to answer your questions or perhaps you start feeling like something is off, you'll be able to compare those findings to your initial assessment and catch changes early.

Of course, you won't perform a thorough neuro assessment on every patient, there's no time for that. However, if your patient presents with a neuro complaint like headaches, motor issues, sensory issues and or altered mental status, they warrant a more thorough detailed neuro exam.

Initial Assessment

- Awake and alert?
  - Do they look at you when you come into the room?
- Are they purposely using their extremities? Are they on their phone using both hands?
- Are they neglecting one side? For example, moving the RUE to assist themselves, but never making an effort to move the left.
- Facial Droop
- Slurring of their speech
- Gaze preference to one side?.

Questions
- Orientation Questions
  - What is their name?
  - Where are you right now?
  - What day, month or year is it?
  - Why are you in the ER?
  - These questions are assessing their ability to think and recall information, and if something is off internally, it will not be easy to do.
- Speech
  - While your patient is speaking, is their speech clear? Slurring?
- Symptoms
  - Always ask the when, how, and where questions.
  - When did the symptoms start?
  - How does the patient describe it.

- Where the symptom is?
- What makes it better and what makes it worse.
- Specific Neuro symptoms include headaches, dizziness, blurry vision, tingling and or numbness, tremors, balance or coordination issues and even bladder and bowel function.
- Ask them if this has ever happened before, and if so what happened. Did it go away on its own or were they diagnosed with something.

Key Point: For thrombolytics, it is essential to know when patients were last normal or when they were last seen normal. Thrombolytics are given within a specific window of 4.5 hours after initial symptom onset, so you have to know when the patient was last seen normal.

- If comatose
  - You can ask ems or family if it was sudden, gradual and intermittent mentation. For example if sudden, it can be from a subarachnoid hemorrhage, if gradual perhaps from a tumor inside the brain, or if fluctuating, perhaps from seizures or other pathologies.
- Trauma
  - Your patient has a headache and keeps passing out, but were just recently hit with a bat to the back of their head, well thats important to know right. Or they recently fell from a ladder, and aren't acting normal per the family.
- Prior medical problems, drugs alcohol and smoking, and current medications. For example, if the patient is on blood thinners, a head bleed may be anticipated after trauma.

Physical Assessment
- GCS
- Pupils
  - Are they equal, round and reactive to light? Is the reactivity to light brisk or sluggish? Are their pupils pinpoint or dilated? What about symmetry? Are they different shapes or sizes from each other? I'll have them follow my finger in a side to side motion, then up and down. Im looking for nystagmus

and whether the patient can actually do it. Ill have them close one eye, focus with the other on my nose, and place fingers in each of the four quadrants, having them tell me how many fingers Im holding up. Ill do this with both eyes.

- Face
  - o Facial Symmetry: Facial Droop
  - o Ask them to smile, and to show their teeth, which makes it easier to see a droop. Ill ask them to lift both of their eye brows up as well.
  - o Sensation: Test for sensation on both sides of the face, asking if it feels the same, or is one less? Or is there tingling or numbness present.
- Upper Extremities
  - o Ask to squeeze your fingers at the same time, noting if strength is equal. Push and pull you, noting symmetry of strength.
  - o Drift: To assess for a drift, I have them close their eyes, lift their arms with palms up, and Ill count to 10 out loud, noting for drift while I'm counting.
  - o Sensation: Touching both sides and asking if it feels the same.
  - o Coordination: Finger to nose test to assess their coordination.
- Lower Extremities
  - o Have them lift against resistance
  - o Push against my palm with pedal flexion and extension.
  - o Drift: Have them lift each extremity separately, and holding for 10 seconds, counting out loud while I note for a drift.
  - o Sensation: Touching both sides and inquiring whether they feel the same or different. If different, how so? Tingling, numb?

Key Point: Become NIH Certified. Crucial to have for taking care of stroke patients.

Neuro Assessment for Intubated Patients

Performing a neuro assessment on an intubated patient comes with challenges as sedative medications prevent an accurate assessment. The challenge lies with, are you going to stop sedation every hour? Most likely not.

- Although you may not be stopping the sedation hourly, keep track of your patients neuro status trends
- If at any point, you detect a change is occurring, you must stop the sedation to obtain an accurate neuro assessment

Physical Assessment

- Pupils
- GCS
- Extremity Assessment
    - Although the pt may not follow commands as a result of the sedation, you can provide a noxious stimuli to assess sensation and motor response
- Noxious Stimuli
    - Withdrawal or localization from the noxious stimuli lets us know sensation is present and movement of the extremity signals that motor function is intact
- Facility Protocol:
    - You need to verify with your own facility what is acceptable as a noxious stimuli, whether nail bed pressure or a trapezius pinch are okay, or whatever your facility finds acceptable.

Key Point

- If you get report from another nurse, do a bedside assessment with them, at least going over the deficits present so you are fully aware of what they are. Anything can happen at any time, and even in the first few minutes after you take report, a patient can stroke out again, and if you dont know what deficits they already had, you may not catch it.
- Finally, dont be afraid to ask another nurse or provider for their opinion. If you feel something is off but cant quite figure it out, do

not hesitate to ask for assistance. Again, time is brain. The important thing is that you recognized something was off.

Gastrointestinal Assessment

Among GI Emergencies, we need to be very vigilant for anything ruptured or perforated as it will lead to massive bleeding as GI tissues are very vascular and infection. For example, a ruptured appendix, gallbladder, spleen, or even ectopic pregnancy. Or Perforated bowel from an Ulcer or severe obstruction.

Some of my busiest patients have been severe GI bleeds, where I've had to give 10+ units of RBC's in the ER to keep them alive before getting permanent surgical interventions.

Keeping emergencies in mind, a quick tip is that you should give extra attention when assessing elderly patients with abdominal pain, as often, their abdominal pain can be from a life threatening condition if left unattended.

Visual Inspection

- Is the abdomen round and distended? (Cirrhotic?)
- Any bruising around the umbilicus or the flanks? Intraperitoneal or retroperitoneal bleeding
- Scars, masses or hernias?
  - **Prior abdominal surgeries increase the risk for Bowel obstructions**
- Patient Position
  - For example, if they are in a fetal position, it can be a sign of peritonitis as stretching out causes irritation and pain.
- Appearance: Are they pale or jaundice? Awake and alert or perhaps stuporous or comatose?

Again, to reiterate, first begin by looking at your patient and their abdomen. This should take no more than a few seconds.

Questions

- Where is the pain?
- Does it radiate?

- When did the part start?
- What were you doing when it started? Was it after eating? What did you eat?
- What makes it worse? What makes it better?
- Describe your pain
  - Intermittent or constant
- Fever
  o Although, you will get a temperature as part of your assessment, still ask your patient if they had a fever at home and or chills, which can point the team in the direction of a possible infection.
- Next, ask if this has ever happened before.
  o There will be times, when your patient has been diagnosed with something, which might be the reason for their symptoms, but wont tell you until you explicitly ask about it.
- Ask about alcohol use? As it puts patients at an increased risk for Liver and pancreatic issues, for cancer, ulcers, and a plethora of other issues.
- As with any other patient, ask about past medical history, surgical history, drug use, smoking history, and any current medications they may be on. Do remember that chronic nsaid use can place patients at an increased risk for stomach ulcers.

Associated Symptoms

- Nausea, vomiting diarrhea and constipation
- For vomiting and diarrhea, ask, how many times per day? What color? Is your patient dehydrated? The color from vomit and stool is important. For example, is it black? Or very dark? Or bright red? These signal the possibility for a GI bleed. Grey stool can be caused by liver and gallbladder issues. Green vomit is bilious in nature, possibly signaling that an obstruction is present. While green or yellowish stool can signal that an infection is present. As for constipation, when was the last bowel movement? And the type of stool? As smalls lumps signal severe constipation. For example,

constipation, nausea and vomiting, combined with abdominal pain, can be caused by an obstruction.

Key Point: If your patient is in the ER for any type of infectious complaint, you must get an oral temp. A temporal temp is not sufficient. And for peds, especially those younger than 1 year old, you need to obtain a Rectal temp. Of course, check with our facility if this is protocol there, and also, of course, explain to the parents why it is necessary.

Moving on, although we are discussing Gastrointestinal issues, I want to make sure you are also asking about **problems with urination.**

- A a kidney infection, or kidney stone, or even a UTI, can manifest as abdominal pain. So ask your patient if there are any issues with urination. Any discharge from their genitalia. Or scrotal pain? As in men, testicular issues can manifest first as lower abdominal pain.

For women of child bearing age:

- Is there a chance of pregnancy?
- Ask about their menstrual cycle, when was the last one? Any issues with it? Are they regular or irregular? You ask to assess for possibility of an ectopic pregnancy, among many other gynecological issues. Of course, you must obtain a pregnancy test on any women of childbearing age who presents with abdominal pain. **Its a cardinal ER rule.**

So here I briefly wanted to talk about how the location of the pain in the abdomen can signal the cause of it. Here, on the right, I have a drawing of an abdomen, which is divided into RUQ, LUQ, RLQ,LLQ, and Epigastric, Right and Left Flank, and suprapubic regions.

- RUQ: Pain in the RUQ, can signal the possibility for liver and gallbladder issues, or even pneumonia in the RLL as the pain can radiate down to the abdomen.

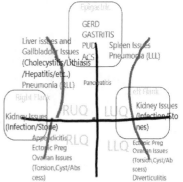

- Epigastric: Pain in the epigastric region can be as a result of Gerd, gastritis, peptic ulcer disease, pancreatitis and even acute coronary syndrome.
- Lower Quadrants: Pain as a result of an ectopic pregnancy, ovarian issues like torsion, and even testicular issues can present as pain in the lower abdomen or suprapubic region.
- RLQ: Appendicitis is common.
- LLQ: Diverticulitis
- Flanks: Kidney issues, like infections and stones.

One thing to keep in mind, is that the location of the pain will not always correlate with the organs in the area. Due to the innervations of the abdomen, pain is often referred. For example, the source of the pain can be on the Right side, but the pain itself may only be present on the Left. So be thorough with your assessments. There's also conditions that cause diffuse abdominal discomfort, like DKA.

Physical Assessment
You are not a GI attending, so keep it simple and stick to the basics.
When palpating, use your whole hand, not just jab with your fingers.
- You're simply looking for areas of tenderness, rigidity, masses or abnormalities.
- For example, is their abdomen soft, flat, nontender and nondistended, or is it firm and rigid, tender and or distended.
- While palpating, keep in mind, the location of the discomfort so you can correlate it with potential causes, so you can ask even more narrow questions and or focus your assessment more.

I wanted to briefly touch on the work up of a GI complaint. For potential liver or gallbladder issues, liver function tests will be ordered by the provider, and these include ALT, AST, bilirubin and albumin, among others. An ultrasound is also commonly ordered for patients with RUQ pain to assess the gallbladder. For pancreatic potential issues, a lipase will be ordered. A cbc will help with seeing if an infection is present, or whether the patient has a low hemoglobin. A bmp will give us lab values to assess kidney health, and electrolytes, which if the patient has severe diarrhea and or vomiting, must be assessed. Urine tests will often be ordered to assess for possible infections and kidney function, among other things. Pregnancy testing to potential eval for an ectopic pregnancy or other gynecological issues. Ultrasound for RUQ pain, and at bedside by providers to quickly visualize bleeding and organs. Ultrasounds often used for women when assessing gynecological pathologies. Ultimately, CT's as they will provide more in depth imaging.

Nursing Tips

- Obtain a pregnancy test for any women in their child bearing years who presents with abdominal pain. You must also have negative pregnancy test before taking a women to CT. Check with your facility if they allow rapid point of care pregnancy testing done with blood. So simply, instead of using urine, you use the patients blood, which can be obtained when you drew their labs or by prickling like you would to check a blood sugar.
- Obtain an ECG for patients complaining with upper abdominal pain who have significant risk factors for ACS such as being a women or a diabetic or significant alterations in vital signs.
- The last tip I have is to get really good with working a **rapid blood transfuser,** because when GI bleed patients tank, they tank. So be ready.

How to be a safe ER Nurse?

Patient safety should be at the top of your priorities. You do not want to be the reason why someone got hurt. You've heard the saying, do no harm. Being safe also allows you to protect your nursing license.

- From day one, anytime you do anything for your patients, you need to ask yourself, is this safe? Why am I doing this? Do I understand how this is going to help my patient? What are the possible complications?If you do not know the answer to any of these, you need to stop and ask. Ask your preceptor, ask pharmacy, ask your provider, ask another nurse. Again, you want to be safe for yourself and for patients. In the beginning, there will be a big gap in your knowledge, but by asking and experiencing as much as possible, you will little by little build your foundation, and get a sixth sense for when something is wrong. So with any procedure, any medication or any intervention, ask yourself, is this safe and appropriate for my patient?
- Always always always ask your patient for their allergies prior to giving any medications or even prior to them getting contrast in CT. Even ask about food allergies before you give a patient a tray of food. You want to make sure you are not giving them something that they are allergic to. Again, ask what their allergies are before giving any medications.
- Specific classes of medications you have to be extra careful with include insulins, opioids, blood thinners, blood pressure meds, and any medication that you are giving to a pediatric patient.
- For blood thinners, what is the reason for the medication? Do you need to have baseline coags? Are they going to surgery any time soon? Are they currently bleeding from anywhere? Is it the right dose?
- For insulins, what is the blood sugar? It needs to be recent, no more than 30 minutes old. Is the patient insulin naive? Do you know the onsets and peaks? Do you know how to treat hypoglycemia?
- For bp meds, always check the blood pressure before administering.

- For IV opioids, is it the right dose? Give very slowly. Are they on a monitor? Have they ever had IV opioids before? Is oxygen equipment readily available if needed? Are they elderly and or peds? I always dilute opioids with normal saline so that I can give it slowly and more controlled. (Check compatibility).
- For peds, always double check the dosing with a buddy nurse.

Again, always ask for help if you do not know something or if you feel unsure about anything.

What should a New ER Nurse focus on?

A new ER nurse needs to be proactive with building their foundation. So being proactive means taking charge of your experiences, the patients you get exposed to, reading outside of work, asking questions, and keeping notes.

In the very beginning, you should focus on having a solid understanding of ACLS, PALS, ABC's, common conditions and your assessments which includes what questions you need to be asking. ACLS and PALS are essential in the ER as they involve rhythm issues like vtach, vfib, svt and symptomatic bradycardia just to name a few. They'll also cover respiratory and cardiac arrest, as well as go over airway management, critical care medications like epinephrine and amiodarone, and also the treatments for strokes and acute coronary syndromes.

The ABC's are also extremely crucial as they are essential to assessing and stabilizing sick patients in the ER. So ensure to educate yourself on the components which entail the assessment portion and treatments or maneuvers. And of course, common conditions and assessments for each. These can include chf exacerbation, stemis, pulmonary embolisms, allergic reactions, seizures, and GI bleeds. Familiarize yourself with how they present, the work up, and treatments. Regarding exposure, you need to be hands on as much as possible. I know it can be intimidating, but ask your charge nurse to give you the sickest patients, from newborns to geriatrics, so that you can see the different types of conditions that commonly come through the ER, as well as getting a good hold on critical care patients. This will build your critical thinking, and polish your skills. If there is a sick patient on the unit, if possible, go and help. Think of questions that you can ask your preceptor or look up. Watch all the procedures, whether its chest tube placement, intubations, or even when they are placing drains. Then at the end of each day, you need to review and go over what you learned, and if you have any gaps in knowledge, you need to be looking it up.

Remember, seriously, no question is a dumb question. You are building yourself up. Ask away. That's how you'll improve little by little, by building your knowledge. Try to answer your own question to get you thinking, then ask your preceptor, your educator, or even your provider to ensure you have the right information. Or even looking it up when you get home.

On your days off, if you are able to, I suggest picking up an emergency nursing book, and reading for an hour or so, to ensure you are constantly educating yourself on ER nursing related topics. If you do so, it'll get to the point where you'll see something in real life that you had previously read about, and because of it, you'll have a better understanding of the patho and treatments used. The key is that you are constantly building your ER brain, even if for an hour on your days off. Little by little, things will start to make more sense.

Know that it will take time. It takes approximately a year for things to really start to come together. Around that time is when I've noticed new Nurses feel way more comfortable and confident in themselves. The key thing is to be patient with yourself, but you must be strategic and proactive with your learning and your experiences. Take the time to appropriately build your foundation so that you can be a safe nurse for your patients and for yourself.

Advice you should hear at least once!

Don't get cocky!

- The ER is not forgiving, it will humble you. Cocky newbies are dangerous because they think they know everything, making them more prone to mistakes. These mistakes can end up hurting or killing someone. On top of this, no one wants to teach or help someone who thinks they know everything. You'll be alone in the ER because of this attitude, and that's terrifying. I'm confident that none of you will be like that but I feel like you should at least hear it once from someone.

It's ok to be slow at first! It's ok to feel overwhelmed!

- Becoming a good ER nurse takes time. There is so much to learn. Within the same day you can take care of really sick patients, sick pediatric patients and even have a crash birth in one of your rooms, so it's perfectly normal to feel slow and overwhelmed, because there's going to be so much happening. The important thing will be that every day you are learning something and little by little becoming the nurse you are meant to be. Things that you should work on daily are prioritizing, grouping your care, safely performing skills faster, and your critical thinking. Also, it's okay to cry. It happens. Pick yourself back up, and keep going. Do not get discouraged.

No question is a dumb question!

- I'm serious. You're dealing with people's lives, so if you ever have any doubt or a question about anything, you better ask. If it's a question on a medication, call your pharmacists and ask away, that's why they are there. If it's an order, call that provider and ask them to clarify. Ask your preceptor. Ask the other nurses. Ask your fellow new nurses. Ask until you get an answer.

Trust your gut, try to figure it out, ask for help!

- If you feel like something is wrong, you have that gut feeling, then something is for sure wrong, even if you can't quite pinpoint it. So take it seriously. What I want you to do, is to try and figure it out. Try to put the pieces together. Do a complete assessment, check anything and everything connected to or touching your patient, and try to figure out what is going on, why you have this feeling. This is so that you start developing your nursing problem solving ability. As ER nurses, a lot of times, we just make it work, so by doing this simple thing consistently, you'll build this ability of kinda just making things work. Let's take a simple thing like placing a pulse ox on your patient but it's not reading, figure it out. Is the cord or the monitor not working or do you have to change the site? Try to figure it out. This principle also applies to everything else, for example, what if your intubated patient starts desatting? What are you going to do? Finally of course, ask for help! Yes try and figure it out, but if you can't, especially in those life saving situations, ask for help! And learn from what happens, reflect on it, so that next time it happens to you, you're better able to handle the situation.

It's ok to ask for a different preceptor!

- Sometimes personalities just don't match. I sincerely believe that it's ok to ask for a different preceptor. Advocate for yourself if you need to, it's your training! I don't see this too often as most people who do precept actually enjoy it, but it does happen, so know that it's ok to ask for a different preceptor if it's just not working out. However, just because I said this, it doesn't mean that you ask for a new preceptor just because they are being hard on you, or because they have high standards. You're dealing with people's lives, they better be strict and have high standards. As I said, the ER is not forgiving, it will humble you, and sometimes preceptors just want to make sure you develop a little tough skin before you go out on your own.

Safety is number one!!!

- If you don't know how to do something, ask for help. If you feel unsure, ask. Check patient allergies. Know exactly what medications you are giving, and make sure they are not contraindicated for your patient. Always ask yourself, is this safe for my patient? Doesn't matter if it's you doing something or a doctor, always ask yourself, is this safe for my patient and don't be afraid to intervene.

Teamwork Makes the Dream Work

- The ER is chaotic, it's hectic, there's always something going on. You have to help each other out. It's a team. It's a family. You see so much despair, and death. Patients can be abusive. And a lot of times, there perhaps isn't even enough staff. So how do you get by? You get by with the help of your team, your support system. Help each other out. Seriously, teamwork makes the dream work.

Cardiorespiratory Arrest (Full Arrest): My experiences

Preparing

You typically get some type of warning that a full arrest patient is coming into your room, which gives you time to do a couple of things.

- Supplies and Equipment
    - Crash cart at bedside and have pads ready to be attached.
    - Suction and bag valve mask
    - Glucometer.
    - Pressurized NS bag ready
    - Supplies to connect onto cardiac monitor
    - IV supplies or IO Gun
    - Ultrasound and ECG machine on standby.
- Let essential staff know: ER provider, Respiratory therapy, Registration, Tech's, Fellow Nurses
- Assign roles: who is working the crash cart (getting meds ready and managing the defibrillator), who is starting an IV/IO and giving meds, who is doing CPR, who is connecting the patient onto the pads and cardiac monitor, who is at the airway, and who is checking a blood sugar for you?
    - Typically you will be recording and keeping track of times.
- What to ask your provider during preparation?
    - How often do you want to do Epi and pulse/rhythm checks?
- Know what meds are in the crash cart
    - Epi, Amiodarone, Magnesium, Lidocaine, Bicarb, Calcium Chloride, Dextrose
- Know how to work the defibrillator
    - How to defibrillate
    - How to pace
    - How to cardiovert

Patients Arrives

- Questions for EMS/paramedics
  - When was the last Epi given?
  - What is the approximate overall downtime?
  - How long has CPR been ongoing for? Was there bystander CPR?
  - What has been the patient's rhythm and any shocks?
  - What's the story? What happened? Medical history?
- Ensure pt gets connected onto the pads and cardiac monitor, ensure good CPR is going, ensure IV/IO access is placed, ensure medications are given, ensure rhythm and pulse checks are occurring, ensure defibrillators are happening as indicated, did endtidal get placed on the patient?
  - Its important to ask the provider before hand how often they want epis and pulses/rhythm checks so we can keep track of them. If epi's are every 3 minutes, then you're keeping time on your watch. 30 seconds before 3 minutes are up, say "Epi will be given in 30 seconds," this helps the team know. Then when its due say "Epi is due," or something along those lines.
  - The same with pulse checks if not basing on the endtidal. Say "pulse check in 30 seconds," again it makes the team aware of what is going on.
  - You want to keep track of times, meds and interventions because as the nurse in charge youre gonna get ask, how many epis have we given? Whats the total downtime so far? Etc, so you want to ensure you have that information readily available.
    - Some hospitals do real time charting on their computer, I still like doing it old school on a white piece of paper then go back and chart everything after everything is done.
- If you get asked for the ultrasound, you already have it ready. With the ultrasound, the providers can check for cardiac activity, cardiac

155

tamponade and right heart strain with Pulmonary embolisms among other things.

- Before ceasing efforts, its crucial to check for cardiac activity because the heart can still be functioning but have a very weak pulse that is not palpable.
- Help figure out reversible causes: H's and T's

After: Was Rosc achieved? (Return of Spontaneous Circulation)
- Pressure support: pressors? Fluids? Blood?
- Is Therapeutic Hypothermia indicated?
- ECG?
- Arterial Line
- Central Line
- Intubated for proper oxygenation
  - Foley Cath, OG tube, soft restraints?
- Send a full set of labs as ordered?
- Carry out treatments/interventions ordered
  - Continue treatment of reversible causes
  - Correct electrolyte abnormalities
- Close monitor because the patient can arrest again
  - Keep them on the defib pads, keep the crash cart handy (call for more meds if needed)

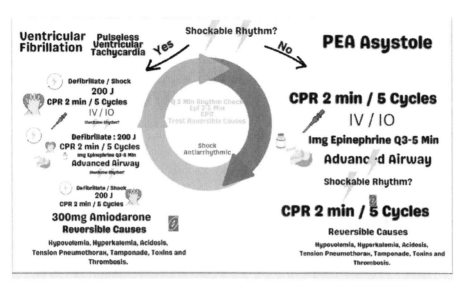

Ventricular Fibrillation **Pulseless Ventricular Tachycardia**

Shockable Rhythm?

Yes

No

PEA Asystole

Defibrillate / Shock
200 J
CPR 2 min / 5 Cycles
IV / IO
Shockable Rhythm?

Defibrillate : 200 J
CPR 2 min / 5 Cycles
1mg Epinephrine Q3-5 Min
Advanced Airway
Shockable Rhythm?

Defibrillate / Shock
200 J
CPR 2 min / 5 Cycles

300mg Amiodarone
Reversible Causes

Hypovolemia, Hyperkalemia, Acidosis, Tension Pneumothorax, Tamponade, Toxins and Thrombosis.

2 Min Rhythm Check
Epi 3-5 Min
CPR
Treat Reversible Causes

Shock
Antiarrhythmic

CPR 2 min / 5 Cycles
IV / IO
1mg Epinephrine Q3-5 Min
Advanced Airway
Shockable Rhythm?

CPR 2 min / 5 Cycles
Reversible Causes

Hypovolemia, Hyperkalemia, Acidosis, Tension Pneumothorax, Tamponade, Toxins and Thrombosis.

Intubations(Rapid Sequence Intubation-RSI): What is our role as the Nurse?

What is Rapid Sequence Intubation? It's an airway management technique where a patient gets sedated then paralyzed, followed by rapid placement of a tube inside their trachea so that a ventilator connected to the tube can breathe for the patient. There are a variety of reasons why a patient can get intubated such as respiratory failure or being unable to protect their airway as with gcs scores less than 8.

The most important aspect of preparing for RSI is preoxygenation. Meaning we place the pt on oxygen in order to build up the oxygen levels within their body, so that while they are being intubated and not breathing, the body has a reserve of oxygen that it can use. So to do this, the gurney should have an o2 tank, attach a regular nasal cannula and crank it up to 6 L and place on the patient, then on the wall oxygen attach a NRB to 15L and place on the patient. **OR** which is more common, get the ambu bag(bag valve mask) and place it over the patients mouth and nose. If the patient is still taking good spontaneous breaths, you simply hold the ambu mask over their mouth and nose, without bagging or squeezing air into them, essentially functioning as a NRB. However, if the patient is not taking their own spontaneous breaths, then yes, you do a 3C tight seal and bag them every 5-6 seconds. You ideally want to preoxygenate for at least a few minutes to build the oxygen up within their body as much as possible.

If the patient is very unstable, including bp and spo2, you'll want to try and address it. If the bp is soft or in other words low, fluids can be administered, but if there is a contraindication to given fluids like CHF, then fluids may be contraindicated or the amount given may be small. Of course, as always, follow what your provider orders. Another way to bring the BP up is a push dose pressor, meaning small doses of epinephrine or phenylephrine, but this is only done by the provider. It's just important for you to know that there are options so you can suggest them if needed.

So all of this is done, including Bp management and preoxygenating, to prevent the pt from tanking during the intubation. Since its more likely to happen if the patient is unstable with a low bp, low spo2, and already acidodic, because after the paralytic is given, the pt is apneic and not breathing, co2 and acids build up, and if you remember from school, acidosis shuts down body processes. Which is why it is very important to prepare in order to prevent any of this from happening.

So now, as far as to equipment, as we've discussed, have suction, nasal cannula, NRB and ambu bags ready. Have your pt on the cm, connected onto spo2, ecg, and bp. Have 1 good working IV, but if you can have 2, even better. Specifically, for the intubation, although the RT and provider usually gather these supplies, you should still know what they are, you'll need a laryngoscope, the blades which are things attached to it, the curved one is called macintosh, the straight one is called a miller blade, you'll also need a stylet which is the blue stick that goes in the ET tube to give it sturdiness while its inserted, and you'll need a co2 detector to confirm placement, its a small square device that gets connected to the et tube after intubation, and it changes color from purple to yellow. Other possible equipment needed is an opa and a glidescope, which is a video assisted laryngoscope.

Post intubation, you'll place a foley to assist with urination and an NG tube to decompress the stomach and prevent acid contents from coming back up. Ensure you check with your facility and or organization for their guidelines and policies, as well as ensure you follow your providers orders, just know that sometimes soft restraints may be placed on patients after they are intubated to ensure that they don't accidentally extubate themselves if a brief moment of wakefulness happens while you are not in the room. Again, ensure you know your policies and guidelines, follow orders, but your preceptor should always be with you. You'll need several IV pumps of course because you'll have your patient on variety of drips for sedation post intubation plus all the other meds for treating your patient. An important question to ask your providers, is what medications will be used for sedation and analgesia prior to intubation, so that these can be prepared and ready once the intubation is successful.

Common sedative medications for intubation include Etomidate,

Ketamine, Propofol and versed, with perhaps etomidate being the most common. Common paralytics include rocuronium and succinylcholine.

Etomidate is hemodynamically stable, meaning it shouldn't affect the patient's vitals directly. Succinylcholine works fast and doesn't last long, while rocuronium can last for an hour. You don't want patients to be paralyzed for so long, but succs can cause hyperkalemia in certain patients so at times Roc is used.

CODE STROKE

Its important for ER nurses to be familiar with stroke protocols because time is brain. Even just a few minutes without perfusion can start causing damage so the faster you can recognize a stroke, the faster your patient gets the necessary treatments. The overall steps of a code stroke include first recognizing stroke like symptoms, activating a code stroke alert, transporting the patient to ct, and ultimately implementing appropriate treatments and interventions. Let's go into some of the details for each step.

So as far as recognition, realizing that the patient is having a stroke, occurs in different ways. The first is out in the field, meaning outside the hospital by EMS. If this happens, they are able to call into the ER, and notify us that a patient who is potentially having a stroke is coming in. This gives us time to get the necessary personnel involved by calling a code stroke ahead of time, you'll hear something along the lines of "Code Stroke Ambulance Bay, ETA 10 minutes." Next, a stroke can be recognized whenever you as an ER nurse are coming into contact with a patient. This includes triage and at any point in their stay. Some facilities want you to get a provider to lay eyes first so they do their own assessment and then call a code stroke, while other facilities want you to call a code stroke as soon as you believe your patient is experiencing a stroke. So make sure you know what your facility does.

Symptoms commonly displayed by stroke patients include facial droop, slurring, or aphasia where your patient can have difficulty understanding or comprehending language, or even difficulty saying what they want to say. Stroke patients can also commonly experience weakness and or numbness on one side of the body, including the face, arms and or legs. They can exhibit drifts, meaning if you ask them to hold their arms or legs up for 10 seconds, the extremity would begin to fall before the 10 seconds were up. Other symptoms can include dizziness and loss of balance, which is common in cerebellar or brainstem strokes. Then of course, vision issues are also common. If your patient is showing any of these symptoms, a code stroke may be activated. Of course, you are new, and it is never wrong to ask a buddy nurse or a provider to come and evaluate the patient if you feel unsure.

As always, it is better to be safe, and if you feel unsure, getting a more experienced nurse is the safest thing to do. But again, make sure you know what your facility does, and of course, while you are new your preceptor should always be with you to ensure you are being and learning how to be safe.

After the code stroke is activated, the most important next step will be getting to CT. However, a lot of things will happen between recognizing the stroke and getting the patient to CT, so lets go over them. The necessary personnel that need to show up include ER providers, neurology, ER nurses, and Radiology, meaning CT needs to make this patient their priority.

Keep in mind that a lot of things happen simultaneously. As with any other patient, the ABC's need to be addressed. For example, if your patient is altered with a gcs of 8 or less and can't protect their airway, you can't go to ct without an established airway, meaning they have to get intubated for airway protection. Another very important thing that must happen is checking a blood sugar, so it needs to be at the top of your to do list, as hypoglycemia can mimic stroke symptoms, and you wouldn't want to be the nurse who gave TPA without checking a blood sugar, that's a pretty big no no.

Next, make sure to hook up the patient to a portable monitor so you can get a set of vitals, as knowing the bp is extremely important for stroke patients.

While all of this is happening, you should also be calling CT to make sure they are ready for the patient. And you should also be working on getting an NIH. The NIH assessment is a standardized way to assess stroke patients for their symptoms, with the higher the number the worse the deficits are so take the time to learn the NIH assessment scale and become certified.

Just as important as getting a blood sugar is going to be asking the patient, their family or ems, when the patient was last seen normal. If the patient woke up with their symptoms, the last seen normal would be when they fell asleep. Its important to ask this question, because tpa can only be giving within 4.5 hours of symptom onset.

As you are heading to ct, you're working on getting a blood sugar, getting a set of vital signs, continuing your neuro assessment and NIH, and obtaining more of the story including medical history and allergies, especially checking for allergies to contrast. If your patient needed to be intubated, that would have been done before going to CT. If time allows, get an IV and get blood work at this time, but you can place the line if one isn't already present between the head ct and the CTA.

So now that your patient made it to CT, they'll get a ct head without contrast. Essentially this is to help differentiate between an ischemic or hemorrhagic stroke. Everything up to this point is the same for both a hemorrhagic and an ischemic stroke. After the initial CT rules out a hemorrhagic stroke, the patient will get a CT Angiogram. Essentially, contrast dye will be injected into the patient to light up the vessels within the brain, so the team can see if there is an obstruction present blocking blood flow, and more importantly where because if its in a large vessel, often called an LVO, or large vessel occlusion, the patient may be a candidate for mechanical thrombectomy where interventional radiology goes in through the vessel, commonly starting at the groin, to remove the clot. As briefly mentioned, you'll place an IV after getting the head ct and get your blood work there, since you need an IV for the CTA. Usually you want an 18 G in the ac, but if you can get an 18 anywhere in the forearm as well, CT usually takes it.

Now lets get into the various treatment methods available for ischemic strokes. You have TPA, a clot buster and thrombectomy, where they go through the femoral arteries to remove the clot using some type of catheter and retrieval device. The main thing to know is that the window for thrombectomy is up to 24 hours, so most facilities still call a code stroke for patients up to 24 hours of last seen normal just in case they are candidates for a thrombectomy, so ensure you know what your facility does. For TPA, the window is 4.5 hours.

Before giving TPA, ensure you have also reviewed the contraindications, as you will be the one administering and must make sure the patient meets the criteria, so that if you have any concerns, they can be voiced and discussed with the team. Ensure consent has been obtained, because TPA has adverse effects that can be deadly, so that patient and the family should at least have an understanding of the risks associated. This is done by the provider, you just have to make sure it happens. Quick tips include placing at least 2 iv's prior to TPA administration if possible, because you don't want to be pocking the patient after giving TPA. Also ensure you have the patients correct weight, as tpa dosing is weight based. Ensure labs have been sent, especially your coags. Know that you will need a second nurse to verify the dosing with you, so ensure you have a buddy nurse there with you. Be prepared to give BP meds prior to administration if needed, and know that your patients who are receiving TPA become 1:1, meaning this patient will be your only patient.

IV Tips

Placing IV's is probably one of the most important skills an ER nurse can have. In any true emergency, medications will need to be given, and for most medications giving them IV means they start working faster, ultimately helping treat the patient faster.

- Know the anatomy! Know where veins are normally supposed to be so that you can look there first.

- Let gravity help you! Let the arm hang a little, ask the patient to squeeze a couple of times. But let gravity help you!

- Don't be afraid to give the vein you see a couple of light taps to get it to pop out more.

- Use a second tourniquet if needed.

- Get an IV catheter and just practice holding it. As well as the motion necessary to advance the catheter into a vein. The more comfortable it feels to hold it and advance, the easier it will be to place an IV in real life.

- Learn how to stabilize veins! They will roll, unless you properly learn how to. Ask your preceptor to review this ! Typically one hand is used for stabilizing, while the other is used for the actual IV placement.

- Practice finding veins on your family and or friends. The skill most needed is learning to recognize how a vein feels, so the more you do it, the more your fingertips get used to it. So when it comes to the real thing, to an actual emergency, you'll be more used to finding good veins.

- Try and try and try again. Even if you're not getting them at first, I promised there's gonna be a turning point where placing IV's kind of just clicks. But you have to put in the work. You should try to place an IV any time you get a chance.

How to give report?

The first thing we have to keep in mind is who are we giving report to? Some ER nurses want a short and sweet report, while others want details, all the details. If it's the ICU or tele, a more thorough report will be required, again they'll want all the details regarding the patient, or at least expect plenty of questions at the end of the report. Hit or miss with medsurg.

Don't forget that its always going to be ok if you say "Hey i'm new, so if I missed anything or you have tips, please let me know, I welcome them!" This can help you relax and at the same time let the other nurse know that you are new and not be a harsh critic.

Now lets go directly into giving report. A quick report still has all of the essentials. These include name and age, chief complaint, history, allergies, what's pending and what the plan is for the patient. Will the pt be admitted, discharged, or pending dispo? Dispo essentially just means what is going to happen with the patient, what is the plan.

Now for a more thorough report, we will be essentially doing everything we already talked about but also going into associated symptoms, what was done for the patient in the ER, pertinent labs, meaning not every single lab result but labs pertinent for this patient or those that are out of the ordinary, for example if a pt came in for chest pain, you must talk about troponins, whether they are positive or negative, and if needed, when the repeats are. Next go into IV sites, their gauge and if any medications are currently infusing. Then go into a current assessment of the patient, giving the last vital signs, and giving the patients aao and gcs status, then respiratory status. You can say " pt is aaox4, gcs 15, c resp e/u at this time." It is important to state if you gave medications like benzo's and at what time, especially since it can make a pt drowsy and appear altered. You'll give the code status, mention if the patient has a foley, an ng tube, a chest tube, ostomy, wounds, a dialysis fistula, or a pacer or defibrillator or even an amputation. If the patient has to be NPO mention it, especially the reason. Go over the allergies, and past medical history. When and which meds are due on their shift?

If the patient is more critical, state which pressors the patient is on and the rate, if intubated mention the size and length of tube, mention which sedation the patient is on and how they are tolerating it, if on bipap mention the settings and if the patient is tolerating the mask. If the patient has a central line, mention the location and type.

You can see the difference in reports, although both include the essentials, one can be quick and concise, while the other goes into pretty much everything.

At the end of the day, take a deep breath, know that its going to be ok, and the more you do it, the easier it'll be for you. Remember to go with the flow, give thorough reports and little by little you'll figure out who wants what, and don't worry if you miss something, that is why at the end they are supposed to ask questions!

Also do your best to give bedside reports! so it is clear to your patients that you are leaving and someone else is assuming care. It's also very important to give a bedside report because anything can happen at any time, and if it happens in between you giving report and the oncoming nurse going in the room, they may blame it on you. Neuro patients require you do an assessment together for the same reason so as to say nothing has changed. Just remember to write in your nursing notes, "Report was given to So and so." I have coworkers who will also add "questions and concerns addressed, no acute change to pt status."

Starting the Day with Critical Patients

If I know I'm getting the critical patients, before getting report, I'll walk by their rooms and take a quick glance. Noting if they are intubated, if the sedation is working appropriately, taking a quick look at the vitals, at how many meds are hanging, and looking at the patient. Is the patient in any distress? Like are they having noticeable airway or breathing problems, are they guarding, are they pale, or are they completely sedated if intubated. Ill also take a quick look at the room, noting anything that may give me clues as to what happened to the patient. If the crash cart is out, I know the patient was very sick. If i see blood tubing, I know the patient got transfused. Essentially taking a quick look to gather clues.

For me, when it comes to critical patients, I prefer having bedside report. I feel like its much safer because I get a more complete report, meaning all the crucial points that need to be communicated are passed onto me. And i'm able to ask any question about anything I see right there and then. For example, with neuro patients, you should do an assessment with the nurse giving you report so that you have a good understanding of their baseline so that later on if something changes, you are very much on top of it. Otherwise, if a change happens in your patient, you may not catch it, and may think it was already their baseline.

After getting bedside report, I typically go one of two ways. If my patients are stable at the moment, I may choose to review their chart. However, if something needs to be done, like lets say your patients bp is tanking, then I will be addressing that first before I do anything else.

If I decide that my patients are stable, i'll quickly review review key parts of their chart. Ill verify the patients chief complaints and admitting diagnosis, Ill review labs and imaging, medical history, allergies to medications, i'll review the patients Medication Administration record, and I'll ensure to review what the plan is for the patient and what is pending so that I can start planning how i will get whats pending done. For example, lets say the patient has a ct pending, or repeat labs, or a med to be administered, Ill start planning when

Ill be doing these pending tasks after I have assessed both of my patients, unless whatever is pending is crucial for the patients plan.

Now, if something pressing needs to be addressed, then I will be doing that first. For example, things like your patients Bp tanking, heart rate or rhythm issues, desatting, needing more sedation, or even seizing. Or even needing to go to CT at that moment because the results could change the management of the patient.

So you did your initial impression, got a bedside report, addressed any issues that needed to be addressed, and are now going to be in the room. So what now? Well, if my patient is stable, I'll start with taking a look at the vitals and familiarizing myself with their ecg rhythm. I'll review all of the medications they have infusing ensuring the pump was programmed correctly and ensuring it is the right med and at some point looking at the MAR and making sure there are orders for the meds. I'll look at the ET tube, looking at the size and length, as well as the vent settings, and if the patient is synchronous with the vent. I'll look again at the sedation so I know which meds and what rates they are going at. I'll assess the patients' access sites whether Iv's, central lines, arterial lines, chest tubes etc. I'll take a look at the og tube, ensuring it is secure and noting the length. i'll look at the urinary catheter ensuring it is in a good position, not kinked, as well as the patient's urine looking for cloudiness or changes in color, and I'll ensure the patient has soft restraints in place if intubated, as well as ensuring there is an order, and assessing the extremities to ensure the soft restraints are not too tight or causing damage.

You'll get to the point where you do everything just mentioned plus your physical assessment simultaneously. Just ensure you spend a little extra time assessing the reason why your patient is there. For example, if CHF exacerbation, listen to their lungs and heart, note their work of breathing, take a look at the spo2, bp and ecg rhythm, note if they have edema, check their cap refill and pulses. Key things though are that you are going to have to be very throughout with your intubated patients, because they cannot communicate back with you. So your initial assessment is very important, so that you have a good baseline to compare to for the rest of the shift. Like always, maintain patient privacy, just ensure you are assessing everything that needs to be assessed, like if there is a femoral central line, you need to assess the site to ensure it is not overtly bleeding causing a big hematoma, or if the patient has a gi bleed or any gastrointestinal issue, ensure to lift the gown and visualize their abdomen.

Common Conditions to really Familiarize yourself with!

Cardiac

- Acute Coronary Syndrome(Stemi, Nstemi, Unstable Angina), CHF, SVT, Bradycardia (Sinus, Junctional, Blocks-1st, 2nd type 1, 2nd type 2, and third degree block), Atrial fibrillation RVR, Atrial flutter, Vtach, Vfib, Hypertensive Emergency, Cardiac Tamponade, Aortic Dissection, Thoracic and Abdominal Aneurysms, and Cardiac Arrest

Respiratory

- Asthma & Copd Exacerbation, Pulmonary Embolism, Pneumonia, ARDS, Pneumothorax, Hemothorax

Neurological

- Stroke (Hemorrhagic/Ischemic), Brain Bleeds (Different Types), Seizures, Meningitis, Encephalitis, Headaches (Different Types), and Bells Palsy

Gastrointestinal

- GI bleed (Upper and Lower), Cholecystitis/Cholelithiasis, Bowel Obstructions, Pancreatitis, Liver failure and cirrhosis, mesenteric ischemia, peritonitis, and GERD

Genitourinary

- Renal Failure(AKI vs CKD-Dialysis), Nephrolithiasis, pyelonephritis, STI's, UTI's, Priapism, Epididymitis, Ectopic Pregnancy, Ovarian and Testicular Torsion, Eclampsia and Preeclampsia, Placental Abruption, Fetal Death

Psych

- Suicidal Ideation and Homicidal Ideation, Depression, Schizophrenia, Bipolar Disorder and **Interventions for Violent patients**

Endocrine

- Diabetic Ketoacidosis, Alcoholic Ketoacidosis, Hypoglycemia, Thyroid Storm, Diabetes Insipidus and SIADH, Myxedema Coma

Other important Conditions

- Anemia, Cancer Complications, DIC, Rhabdomyolysis, Sickle Cell Crisis, Etoh Withdrawals and Delirium Tremens, Etoh Intoxication, Opioid Overdose and illicit drug overdoses, Burns

Shock States

- Anaphylactic, Cardiogenic, Obstructive, Septic, Hypovolemic, Neurologic

Top 10 Clinical Skills you need to master!

1. IV placement and Blood Draw
2. Taking ECG's
3. Intramuscular Injections
4. Using a defibrillator
   a. Knowing how to defibrillate, cardiovert and pace
5. Using a Rapid Blood Transfuser and Administering Blood Products
6. Using Central Lines, Arterial Lines, Porticaths, and Picc Lines
7. Placing a urinary catheter and Nasogastric tube
8. Managing an Intubated Patient, chest tubes, and EVD
9. Placing Restraints
10. Placing oxygen (NC, NRB, AMBU Bag) and giving basic breathing treatments
    a. Inserting OPA/NPA

Legal Issues to familiarize yourself with

HIPPA, Holds & Restraints ,Mandated Reporter, DNR/DNI-POLST, Emtala, Consents, Minors, Battery

Must Know Numbers

Charge Nurse, Provider, RT, Security, CT, MRI, XRAY, Ultrasound, Registration

Certifications you need to get! (Courses)

ACLS, PALS, BLS, NIH Stroke Scale, CEN (Certified Emergency Nurse), ENPC(Emergency Nursing Pediatric Course), TNCC (Trauma Nursing Core Course), ED Triage Course

Scavenger Hunt: Know Where Things Are At!

Equally as important as everything else, you should be familiar with the location of several things in your emergency department. These can include the crash carts, ECG machines, pyxis, warming/cooling devices, glucometer, IV pumps, rapid blood transfuser, seizure pads, ultrasound machines, ventilators, portable glidescope, I/O gun and the supply room. (Perhaps the most important are the restrooms!) In the supply room, know where respiratory equipment is, restraints, supplies for central lines, arterial lines and chest tubes. Know where the foleys are, where the NG tubes are. Where code brown supplies are.

Sometimes, pyxis will not have the same medications, so if so ensure you know which pyxis has which medications.

I also recommend knowing where CT, Ultrasound, MRI and Lab are. As well as the different departments of your organization/hospital. If your ER is in charge of some part of the "Code Team," figure out where the 'backpack' is with all the supplies and what's in it.

Know where pediatric supplies are if kept separately.

Staying organized: The Brain

Below is how I stay organized with each patient. I typically grab a white blank sheet of paper, fold it in half, and note the sections below. It is important to stay organized because you will have multiple patients at a time and you need to know what each patient is there for, what's pending, their allergies and so forth.

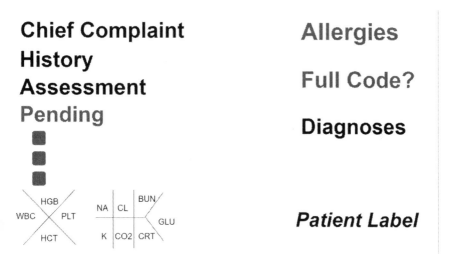

This is a simple example of how it would look for a chest pain patient.

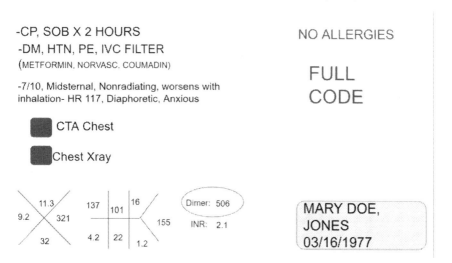

Practice Questions

1. Out of the rhythms listed below, which one requires immediate defibrillation?
   A) Supraventricular Tachycardia
   B) 3rd Degree AV Block
   C) Ventricular Fibrillation
   D) Ventricular Tachycardia with a Pulse

2. Which medication is typically given every 3-5 minutes in cardiac arrest?
   A) Amiodarone
   B) Epinephrine
   C) Magnesium Sulfate
   D) Lidocaine

3. Out of the rhythms listed below, which one requires immediate synchronized cardioversion?
   A) Ventricular Fibrillation
   B) Unstable Supraventricular Tachycardia
   C) Stable Chronic Atrial Fibrillation
   D) Sinus Bradycardia

4. When performing synchronized cardioversion, we MUST select the sync option, what does it synchronize to?
   A) R wave of ECG
   B) P wave of ECG
   C) T wave of ECG
   D) Q wave of ECG

5. What age and below do we not administer NSAIDS to (Ibuprofen etc)?
   A) < 1 year
   B) <6 months
   C) <10 years
   D) <9 months

6. What is the typical dosing for Ibuprofen in children?
   A) 10 mg/kg
   B) 15 mg/kg
   C) 5 mg/kg
   D) 2.5 mg/kg

7. What is the typical dosing of Adenosine in ACLS for SVT?
   A) 5mg, 12mg, 12mg
   B) 8mg, 10mg, 12mg
   C) 6mg, 12mg, 12mg
   D) 10mg, 15mg, 20mg

8. In rapid sequence intubation, is the sedative or paralytic given first?
   A) Paralytic is given first
   B) Sedative is given first
   C) Both are given at the same time

9. What is the most commonly used sedative in Rapid Sequence Intubation?
   A) Propofol
   B) Etomidate
   C) Ketamine
   D) Versed

10. Why do we preoxygenate prior to Rapid Sequence Intubation?
    A) To help ease patient discomfort
    B) To help increase oxygen reserves
    C) To help facilitate ET tube passage
    D) To help prevent blood pressure from dropping

11. What is the typical dosing of Acetaminophen in children?
    A) 10 mg/kg
    B) 15 mg/kg
    C) 5 mg/kg
    D) 20 mg/kg

12. What is the lowest score a patient can receive on the Glasgow Coma Scale?

  A) 1
  B) 15
  C) 5
  D) 3

13. Phenytoin needs what prior to administration?

  A) A large bore IV in the AC
  B) Filter
  C) Sodium level checked prior to
  D) Vigorous Shaking

14. Why is 3% hypertonic saline typically given in cerebral edema?

  A) To help increase cerebral blood flow
  B) To help prevent seizures
  C) To help with sodium imbalances
  D) To help reduce intracranial pressure

15. What is the purpose of PEEP in mechanically intubated patients?

  A) Helps improve gas exchange
  B) Helps prevent barotrauma
  C) Helps reduce FIO2 required
  D) Helps recruit and maintain alveoli

16. What medication is typically given in Torsades De pointes?

  A) Epinephrine
  B) Amiodarone
  C) Lidocaine
  D) Magnesium

17. What is the typical treatment of a tension pneumothorax in the ER?

  A) Rapid Sequence Intubation
  B) High Flow Oxygen
  C) Needle Decompression and Chest Tube Placement
  D) BIPAP

18. What is the most common first line treatment for an asthma exacerbation?
   A) Bipap
   B) Magnesium
   C) Steroids
   D) Albuterol

19. In patients with suspected opioid overdose, what is the reversal agent?
   A) Atropine
   B) Protamine Sulfate
   C) Naloxone
   D) Lactated Ringer's Bolus

20. What parameter do we typically titrate vasoactive medications to?
   A) SBP
   B) ICP
   C) MAP
   D) CPP

21. What is the main medication used for anaphylactic shock?
   A) Benadryl
   B) Epinephrine
   C) Solumedrol
   D) Famotidine

22. What are the first line common medications used for Atrial Fibrillation with a Rapid Ventricular Response?
   A) Lidocaine and Amiodarone
   B) Magnesium and Digoxin
   C) Amiodarone and Metoprolol
   D) Diltiazem and Metoprolol

23. What two main side effects do we closely monitor for when a patient is receiving propofol?
   A) Headaches and Flushing
   B) Respiratory Depression and Hypotension
   C) Arrhythmias and Chest Pain
   D) Potassium Imbalances and Renal Impairment

24. Why do we tend to use propofol as a sedative for intubated neuro patients?
A) Slow onset and long duration
B) Fast Onset and short duration
C) Easier to titrate
D) Does not require a central line

25. What is the antidote used in acetaminophen overdose patients to help prevent liver damage?
A) Flumazenil
B) Naloxone
C) Protamine Sulfate
D) Acetylcysteine

26. Which insulin can be given intravenously?
A) Humulin N
B) NPH
C) Regular (Humulin R)
D) Long Acting Lantus

27. Why is an ECG obtained within 10 minutes of arrival for patients presenting with chest pain?
A) To rule out myocardial ischemia or damage
B) To rule out a tension pneumothorax
C) To rule out respiratory conditions
D) To ensure a baseline ECG is recorded

28. What are the most common symptoms seen with an exacerbation of congestive heart failure?
A) Wheezing and Dyspnea
B) Increased Urination, Thirst and Appetite
C) Dyspnea and Peripheral Edema
D) Confusion and Shakiness to hands

29. In a CHF exacerbation, which medication will help decrease preload and afterload?

A) Furosemide

B) Nitroglycerin

C) Aspirin

D) Morphine

30. In STEMI patients, besides the ECG, what is another important initial step in their care?

A) Obtaining a troponin level

B) Administering Aspirin

C) Obtaining a chest xray

D) Administering Nitroglycerin

31. What is the preferred definitive treatment of a STEMI patient?

A) Primary Percutaneous Coronary Intervention (PCI)

B) Fibrinolytic Therapy

C) Coronary Artery Bypass Grafting

D) Aspirin Administration

32. What is the time frame window to administer a thrombolytic in strokes?

A) Within 3 hours

B) Within 8 hours

C) Within 4.5 hours

D) With 24 hours

33. At what ICP level do we typically start considering more invasive measures like Hypertonic Saline (23.4%) and Mannitol?

A) 20 mm Hg

B) 15 mm Hg

C) 10 mm Hg

D) 25 mm Hg

34. What is the preferred Benzodiazepine for active seizures without IV access? To be administered IM.
   A) Lorazepam
   B) Midazolam
   C) Diazepam
   D) Clonazepam

35. What condition can occur if hyponatremia is correctly too rapidly?
   A) Marfan Syndrome
   B) Rheumatoid Arthritis
   C) Kawasaki Disease
   D) Osmotic Demyelination Syndrome

36. What is the typical first line antihypertensive medication used in patients who will be receiving a thrombolytic for a stroke?
   A) Nitroglycerin
   B) Metoprolol
   C) Labetalol
   D) Propofol

37. What medication is typically used as a drip to control BP in brain bleeds?
   A) Labetalol
   B) Nicardipine
   C) Verapamil
   D) Propofol

38. What is the typical SBP desired in brain bleeds?
   A) Around 140
   B) Around 150
   C) Around 130
   D) Around 160

39. What type of brain bleed is most commonly seen with a ruptured aneurysm?
   A) Subdural
   B) Epidural
   C) Subarachnoid
   D) Intracerebral

40. Out of the list below, which is a contraindication for BIPAP?

A) Decreased Mentation

B) Normal Spo2

C) Unable to obtain IV access

D) Crackles to Lung Fields

41. Which vasopressor is a pure alpha agonist?

A) Epinephrine

B) Dobutamine

C) Dopamine

D) Neosynephrine

42. What is the typical first medication used for symptomatic bradycardia?

A) Atropine

B) Dobutamine

C) Dopamine

D) Metoprolol

43. During a cardiac arrest, do you defibrillate PEA or Asystole?

A) Yes

B) No

C) Depends on patient presentation

D) Provider preference

44. If you as the nurse anticipate a CTPA to help rule out a pulmonary embolism, what size and site should you attempt to place the IV?

A) 18 G in the hand

B) 20 G in the AC

C) 18 G in the AC

D) 22 G in the forearm

45. What lab value is useful in ruling out a Pulmonary Embolism or DVT?

A) Lactate

B) D-Dimer

C) INR

D) BNP

46. What medication is typically used to relieve nausea?

A) Ondansetron

B) Sodium Bicarbinate

C) Haldol

D) Magnesium

47. What is the most appropriate initial way to provide high levels of oxygen for patients presenting with respiratory distress including tachypnea and accessory muscle use?

A) Bag Valve Mask

B) Nasal Cannula

C) Non Rebreather Mask

D) ET Tube

48. Which of these is NOT a contraindication for thrombolytic therapy?

A) Recent Intracranial Hemorrhage

B) Ischemic Stroke within 3 months

C) SBP 220s

D) Hx of Diabetes Mellitus

49. In critical patients with a pulmonary embolism where thrombolytics failed to significantly improve symptoms, what is another treatment available?

A) Thrombectomy

B) PCI

C) Heparin Infusion

D) Rapid Sequence Intubation

50. What two vasopressors can be given as push doses by providers in emergencies?

A) Levothyroxine and Norepinephrine

B) Dobutamine and Dopamine

C) Phenylephrine and Epinephrine

D) Vasopressin and Dopamine

51. What is important to check in patients who are altered?
   A) DNR status
   B) Point of Care Glucose
   C) Family History
   D) Suicidal Ideation

52. When a patient is suspected to be septic as shown by presentation and vital signs, how soon should antibiotics be administered to improve outcomes?
   A) Ideally within 1 hour
   B) Ideally within 3 hours
   C) Ideally within 6 hours
   D) Ideally within

53. What does Source Control mean when caring for patients with sepsis?
   A) Prevent hospital acquired infections
   B) Locate and treat the source
   C) Provide adequate fluid resuscitation
   D) Avoid vasopressor use

54. Family brings a patient into the ER for sudden onset headache, vomiting, and neuro deficits after striking his head yesterday. What diagnostic study would be best to prioritize as the nurse when caring for the patient to assess for intracranial hemorrhage?
   A) Chest Xray
   B) MRI of the head
   C) CT of the head
   D) Ultrasound

55. A patient presents with an expanding intracranial hemorrhage after falling. The patient is currently on warfarin. What are the reversal agents for warfarin?
   A) Vitamin K, PCC, FFP
   B) Protamine Sulfate and Flumazenil
   C) Narcan and Activated Charcoal
   D) Fomepizole and Acetylcysteine

56. What electrolyte in DKA is typically affected and should be monitored closely for arrhythmias?
 A) Sodium
 B) Magnesium
 C) Phosphate
 D) Potassium

57. Which of the following is not considered when determining if DKA has resolved?
 A) Anion gap less than 15
 B) Bicarb greater than 18
 C) Controlled glucose level
 D) Normal range of potassium

58. Why is intubation typically avoided unless absolutely necessary in DKA patients?
 A) Ventilator may be unable to keep up with respiratory rate and tidal volume
 B) Visualizing vocal cords is typically more difficult in DKA patients
 C) Unable to obtain consent since patients are commonly altered
 D) To prevent hospital acquired pneumonia

59. Which of these medications is typically not used for hyperkalemic patients?
 A) Insulin and Dextrose
 B) Calcium Gluconate
 C) Sodium Bicarbonate
 D) Lidocaine

60. What class of medications are commonly used to treat alcohol withdrawal and delirium tremens?
 A) Benzodiazepines
 B) Cephalosporins
 C) SSRI's
 D) Alpha Blockers

Answers

1.C 2.B 3.B 4.A 5.B 6.A 7.C 8.B 9.B 10.B 11.B 12.D 13.B 14.D 15.D
16.D 17.C 18.D 19.C 20.C 21.B 22.D 23.B 24.B 25.D 26.C 27.A 28.C
29.B 30.B 31.A 32.C 33.A 34.B 35.D 36.C 37.B 38.A 39.C 40.A 41.D
42.A 43.B 44.C 45.B 46.A 47.C 48.D 49.A 50.C 51.B 52.A 53.B 54.C
55.A 56.D 57.D 58.A 59.D 60.A

Tips for 12 Hour Shifts and Thriving as a Nurse

- Develop resilience and essentially learn to be unbothered. Your coworkers, at times, will be stressed. Your patients will be in pain. As a result, rude comments or remarks may be said or something along those lines. Don't take it personal. The only thing you have control over is how you react, so be unbothered and let it go.
- You MUST have good shoes and use compression socks if you can. You will walk multiple miles per day and at times may minimally sit down. Good shoes and compression socks will help prevent your feet from hurting. You need to go to a store where your gait and pressure points on your feet are assessed and buy good shoes based on recommendations.
- When you are working multiple days in a row, you need a routine to stick to. Get home, eat something light if needed, shower, and get ready for bed. If needed a few minutes of mindless scrolling. But you need to sleep at least 7 hours. If not, you find yourself less alert, more irritable, more stressed and prone to aches.
- Foster a sense of team work makes the dream work environment. Help your coworkers so that they help you in return. You will spend a lot of time with coworkers so why not help make your department more of a family.
- Keep good posture and relax your shoulders when charting. Don't bend or lift with your back. Elevate the bed to your height or get a stool to sit on. Try and sit often when possible to give your feet a break. Don't stand in one place with knees locked for a long time.
- Take your mandated breaks. Ideally go somewhere off the unit. If possible, elevate your feet while you eat. Try to get your mind off work related issues during breaks, even a bit of mindless scrolling can help.
- Although I love being an ER Nurse, the beauty of nursing is how flexible it is. Hate your department? Switch to a new one. Hate the unit you're in? Switch to a new one? Don't want to work in the

hospital? Go outpatient. Public health. Home health. Urgent care. Case management. So forth.

- General tips: Exercising and stretching regularly help prevent injuries. Be mindful of not doing so much overtime that it burns you out. Massages with a good masseuse are life saving. Good sleep is essential so don't cheap out on a mattress. Enjoy life outside of work.

BE PROACTIVE, NOT REACTIVE

As an ER nurse you should be **Proactive, Not Reactive.** You should prepare for critical patients ahead of time. Your rooms should have a bag valve mask, suction, supplies to connect a patient onto a cardiac monitor and supplies needed to place an IV and so forth should be readily available. IV pumps and poles if the gurney does not come with one should also be readily available. Your point of care glucose monitor should be checked as soon as you get onto the unit to ensure that it's ready when it's needed. **There is always something to do.**

If your patient is going to get intubated, you know that they'll need a urinary catheter, an OG tube, and possibly soft restraints, so if you're free get the supplies. You know that you'll need sedation medications for after the fact, so get them ready.

If you anticipate a patient needing fluids, spike the bag. If you anticipate pressors, mix them and have them ready. If you anticipate a central line, gather the supplies and have them ready. Same for Arterial lines, chest tube placement and even a paracentesis.

Whatever your patient is there for, you can prepare and be proactive by asking yourself, **"What are some of the complications?"** And **"How can I monitor them?"** For example, your patient came in GCS 3 related to an opioid overdose requiring narcan. What are some complications? Well, the patient's mentation and respiratory status can again begin to decline if the narcan starts to wear off which if not caught can lead to respiratory arrest. So how can we monitor them? You could be at the bedside keeping an eye on them, watching for equal chest rise and fall. Well what if you have several other patients to care for? What now? What about endtidal co2? It can be very useful in monitoring your patients.

Again, there is always something to do. **Be Proactive, Not Reactive.**

Please reach out!!

If you have any questions regarding anything emergency nursing, please reach out! Such as why a certain intervention was done for your patient, or if after attempting to review you aren't understanding a topic or even if you need advice regarding anything emergency nursing, please reach out to me at Emergencychaos@gmail.com with the Subject "Question for Emergency Chaos." In return, I ask you please leave a review for the book and attach a screenshot to the email. **Please do not hesitate to reach out!!**

Thank you so much for your time and support.

Welcome to the ER.

THE MORE YOU KNOW, THE SAFER A NURSE YOU ARE!
Check out our other books!

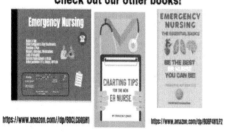

https://www.amazon.com//dp/B0CLCG0GH1

https://www.amazon.com//dp/B0CPJY4S72

https://www.amazon.com/dp/B0BF4R3J2

Made in United States
Troutdale, OR
01/03/2025

27545595R00106